ON DIVORCE

The Library of Conservative Thought
Russell Kirk, Series Editor

Burke Street, by George Scott-Moncrieff.

The Case for Conservatism, by Francis Graham Wilson.

*Collected Letters of John Randolph of Roanoke to
John Brockenbrough, 1812-1833*, edited by Kenneth Shorey.

A Critical Examination of Socialism, by William Hurrell Mallock.

Edmund Burke: Appraisals and Applications,
edited by Daniel E. Ritchie.

Edmund Burke: The Enlightenment and Revolution, by Peter J. Stanlis.

The Essential Calhoun, by John C. Calhoun.

A Historian and His World, A Life of Christopher Dawson 1889-1970,
by Christina Scott.

I Chose Freedom, by Victor A. Kravchenko.

I Chose Justice, by Victor A. Kravchenko.

On Divorce, by Louis de Bonald.

Orestes Brownson: Selected Political Essays, edited by Russell Kirk.

*The Politics of the Center, Juste Milieu in Theory and Practice, France
and England, 1815-1848*, by Vincent E. Starzinger.

Regionalism and Nationalism in the United States, by Donald Davidson.

The Social Crisis of Our Time, by Wilhelm Roepke.

ON DIVORCE

Louis de Bonald

Translated and edited by

Nicholas Davidson

Foreword by Robert Nisbet

Transaction Publishers
New Brunswick (U.S.A.) and London (U.K.)

Translation of *Du divorce, considéré au XIXᵉ siècle,* third edition (Paris: Le Clère, 1818; original edition 1801)

Library of Congress Catalog Number: 91-14608
ISBN: 0-88738-439-0
Printed in the United States of America

Library of Congress Cataloging-in-Publication Data

Bonald, Louis-Gabriel-Ambroise, vicomte de, 1754–1840.
  [Du divorce, considéré au XIXe siècle.   English]
  On Divorce / Louis de Bonald ; translated and edited by Nicholas Davidson.
    p.   cm.—(The Library of conservative thought)
  Translation of: Du divorce, considéré au XIXe siècle.
  ISBN 0-88738-439-0
  1. Divorce.   2. Family.   I. Davidson, Nicholas, 1955–
II. Title.   III. Series.
HQ814.B6613   1991
306.89—dc20   91-14608
                                                             CIP

CONTENTS

Foreword by Robert Nisbet   vii

The Importance of Bonald   xi

Translator's Note   xxiii

Introduction   3

1   Of the Proposed Civil Code   34

2   Of Domestic Society   42

3   Of Public Society   54

4   Of Marriage   62

5   Of the Three States of Society   67

6   Of Society among the Jews   79

7   Of Society among the Orientals, Greeks, and Romans   85

8   Of Society among Christian Peoples   94

9   Revolution in Christian Society   100

10   Of the French Revolution   105

11   General Considerations on Divorce   108

12   Conclusion   130

Appendix   151

Addendum   167

Summation on the Divorce Question   171

Index   199

FOREWORD

by Robert Nisbet

MUCH is owing Nicholas Davidson for editing and translating Bonald's *On Divorce*. It is the first of Bonald's works to reach English translation, after nearly two centuries, and I hope that this book will encourage others to do likewise, for Bonald left behind him a very considerable number of books and articles. *On Divorce* is one of Bonald's most important works, and Mr. Davidson has done ample justice to it in both his exemplary translation and his sage and cogent introduction.

Bonald was one of that hardy group of thinkers who, at the end of the eighteenth century, formed what has sometimes been called the Anti-Enlightenment. Edmund Burke began it all with his *Reflections on the Revolution in France* in 1790. His book was like a fire bell in the night, awakening or mobilizing thinkers in virtually every Western European country to the iniquity of the French Revolution and of the Enlightenment that preceded it. Others were quick to follow. In 1796 Bonald's *Theory of Political and Religious Power* was published while he was in self-imposed exile from his beloved France. In the same year appeared Joseph de Maistre's *Considerations on France*. Soon after there began a procession of books echoing the basically conservative, even reactionary themes of Burke, Bonald, and Maistre, among them Adam Müller's *Elements of Statecraft* in 1810, Friedrich von Savigny's *A Defense of Historical Tradition in Government*, 1814, Karl Ludwig von Haller's monumental *Restoration of Political Science*, 1816–1834, Hegel's *Foundations of the Philosophy of Law*, 1821, and slightly later in Spain Donoso y Cortés's *On Absolute Mon-*

archy in Spain and Jaime Balmes's *Protestantism Compared with Catholicism.*

Taken together these books, nearly all of which made clear their debt to Burke's great *Reflections* of 1790, constituted a conservative or traditionalist renascence. It was really more than a renascence. It was a fierce insurgency against not only the Revolution in France but the principles regnant in the Enlightenment which the traditionalists saw as the immediate cause of the Revolution. These were principles which, it was believed, had betrayed the great Christian-feudal heritage of Western Europe.

Looking about them in post-Revolutionary Europe, the conservatives saw fragmentation and atomization of what had once been an organically articulated social order. Theirs was the mandate of, not conservation, but restoration of the order that the Jacobins had sought to devastate during the Revolution. These principles had on earlier occasions going back to the Dark Ages saved Europe from the ravages of alien invaders; there was no reason, the conservatives believed, why the basically Christian-feudal principles couldn't again save the West, this time from the ravages of Jacobin zealots of the Revolution, themselves acting under the inspiration of such members of the Enlightenment as Rousseau, Diderot, and d'Alembert, all of whom had detested both feudalism and Christianity.

Bonald was one of the leading lights in Western Europe in this work of restoration. He was an active politician but he was also a thinker of profound character. His deepest respect was for the Europe that had reached its height in the Middle Ages, the Europe of ultramontane Christianity and of common feudal principles that gave political unity to the entire West. Such was Bonald's devotion to the medieval synthesis that he was sometimes called "a prophet of the past" and "the last of the scholastics." He seems to have paid little heed to such characterizations. In truth, it was not a whole epoch of the past he was trying to revive; only some of the constitutive elements of that epoch, starting with family, local community, region, monastery, and other buffers between individual and national state.

The Enlightenment and Revolution had glorified the individual and the state, each conceived abstractly, no longer a part of the larger social order. Philosophes and Jacobins were particularly scornful of all that lay in between individual and state in the way of institutions and communities. Hence the pulverizing legislation of the Revolution directed against patriarchal family, local community, guild, monastery, and other groups and associations intermediate to man and state.

The greatest contribution of Bonald principally but of other conservatives too was the reawakening in Western Europe after the Revolution of an appreciation of these intermediate ties among human beings, with the family and church leading the way. Auguste Comte, founder of systematic sociology, was lavish in his praise of what he called "the retrograde school" and of Bonald specifically, whom Comte credited with actually having founded the science of social statics—that is, of the order-making elements and processes of society. Saint-Simon was also an admirer of Bonald, declaring that it was from Bonald that he had learned most about the composition of "organic periods" in the history of society.

The great Frédéric Le Play, true founder of empirical sociology, especially of the family and local community, was properly characterized by the French critic Sainte-Beuve as "a Bonald revived, progressive and scientific." Even Proudhon, anarchist and enemy of state and church, praised and cited Bonald on the importance of the patriarchal family and its environing institutions.

It was not a conservative but a liberal socialist, Gunnar Myrdal, who in my opinion came closest in his appraisal of the significance of the early conservatives for modern social thought. "The conservative wing," wrote Myrdal, "profited from its 'realism.' In its practical work it abstained from speculating about a 'natural order' other than the one that existed; it studied society as it was and actually came to lay the foundations for modern social science."

Is it likely that the resources of so powerful and wide-ranging a mind as Bonald were used up completely in their impact upon such nineteenth-century figures as Comte, Le Play, and Proudhon and are consequently inutile today? I think not. Some of the deepest problems we face in the social order today are close kin to those Bonald and his fellow conservatives faced in their day. I agree with Nicholas Davidson that that is why "Bonald's thought remains so interesting today. Present at the birth of leftism and rightism alike, he grasps the fundamental issues at stake with an immediacy that would in many cases be hard to replicate."

THE IMPORTANCE OF BONALD

by Nicholas Davidson

IN an age contemptuous of its past and disturbed by its present, the neglect of the former feeds an incomprehension of the latter, and we find ourselves debating the relative merits of recent mediocrities, while ignoring the seminal thinkers who, like perennial springs, continue to determine the courses in which we travel, often without our knowledge.

Surely few such thinkers have been more scandalously neglected than Louis-Gabriel-Ambroise, vicomte de Bonald, whose name is all but unknown at present, to the point that this is the first English translation of any of his major works.

Conservatism is the movement that seeks to counter the forces unleashed in the French Revolution. It is thus not accidental that the three principal founders of conservatism all developed their doctrines in reaction to the Revolution: in England, Edmund Burke; in France, Joseph de Maistre and Louis de Bonald, who had read and admired Burke, but who focused their thought on different areas than the great Whig. Maistre and Bonald are so similar that, for some purposes, they may be considered as a unit, differing largely in style, and not always in that: as Maistre towards the end of his life wrote to Bonald: "I have thought nothing you have not written; I have written nothing you have not thought."[1] As this statement also hints, however, these two allies did not cover exactly the same ground; and consequently, if one wishes to under-

---

[1] Quoted in *De Bonald,* by Henri Moulinié (Paris: Felix Alcan, 1915), p. 59. This is the standard work on Bonald.

xi

stand the nature of conservatism, it is necessary to refer to Burke, Maistre, and Bonald.

Of the three, Bonald seems to have been the originator of the term *conservative* in its modern sense. It is in his work, in contrast to that of Burke, Maistre, and Chateaubriand, that one first encounters the frequent use of the expressions *to conserve* and *conservative*. This usage occurs in Bonald's very first work, *Théorie du pouvoir* ("A Theory of Power"), published in 1796, and in all his subsequent major works. Thus when Bonald and Chateaubriand cofounded the influential journal *Le Conservateur* in 1818, the word was very familiar to Bonald; and it is precisely around 1818 that the habit of contrasting "liberal" and "conservative" sides of the political spectrum seems to have begun. Thus we can, with considerable confidence, attribute the origin of the word "conservative" in its modern sense to Bonald.

The word does not initially have exactly its modern meaning in Bonald, however: it appears on the very first page of *On Divorce,* not in reference to men, but in reference to God, whose will is described as "conservative of created beings." Bonald presumably took the word over from its feudal usage, which is preserved in vestigial form in the title "museum conservator." A "conservator" in medieval Europe was an official charged with the protection of the rights, liberties, and privileges attributed to given categories of persons and institutions: for example, the council of Würzburg in 1287 appointed conservators to protect the privileges of certain religious persons; the University of Paris possessed conservators to protect its academic rights; under Henry V of England, a conservator was appointed for each seaport, "to enquire of all offences done against the king's truce and safe conducts, upon the main sea, out of the liberties of the cinque ports."[2] Thus a conservator's function is to protect existing rights and liberties

[2] *Encyclopaedia Britannica,* eleventh edition (1910), article "Conservator."

and to preserve the peace. It is in a sense approaching this that one must understand the word in Bonald's writings, a meaning eventually extended to those political forces seeking to *conserve* society.

We have, then, already gained two reasons to read Bonald: (1) he was one of the three principal founders of conservatism, which, as one of the central movements of our time, is clearly worthy of scrutiny; (2) he appears to have given the conservative movement its very name.

I believe, however, that there is a more important reason than either of these to read Bonald, and that he has a particular message for modern times. In a political society increasingly fragmented into competing interest groups, in which categories of gender, age, race, and ethnicity are barefacedly turned against each other in pursuit of change and power, we have lost the ability to see society whole. There are no social questions in the modern world anymore, there are only women's questions, blacks' questions, old people's questions, children's questions; at the very best there are family questions; we no longer see the relations between these groups and the workings of society as a whole; and the very movement that, distantly related to that of Bonald, would like to hinder this slide into disintegration no longer knows how to combat this mindset without invoking its terms: if the issue is "affirmative action," the best counter it can muster is "reverse discrimination"; if it is a movement of radical women, the best it can do is a movement of conservative women; if the issue is abortion, the best it can do is children's rights; and, trapped in the dialectic of the forces it would like to oppose, the only significant variable is the speed of its retreat. It is to this that Bonald brings the remedy, a remedy that is sure and decisive, not hard to grasp, and devastating to its antagonist. "It is a fertile source of error," he says in the very first sentence of *On Divorce,* "when treating a question relative to society, to consider it by itself, with no *relationship* to other questions, because society itself is only a group of *relationships."* In the contemplation of this truth lies the effective cure, and the only cure, to the social disintegration that afflicts us, whose advance has hitherto seemed so ineluctable.

It remains to say a few words about the life of this extraordinary personality.

*   *   *

Louis-Gabriel-Ambroise de Bonald was born in 1754 in the town of Millau to a noble family that had been established since the 1300s in the Rouergue region of the south of France. His father died when he was four, and he was brought up largely by his mother, a devout Catholic. The faith she inspired in her young son was never to leave him; indeed, he was in the course of his life to be responsible for several notable conversions, including those of the Swiss philosopher Karl Ludwig von Haller and of Lamartine's mistress, Madame Julie Charles, who is immortalized in Lamartine's poetry. The young Bonald received a rigorous theological, classical, and mathematical education at a school at Juilly run by the Oratorians, who had taken up the slack caused by the expulsion of the Jesuits from France in 1762. He was an exceptional student, and appears to have had some exceptional teachers; his principal teacher, Fr. Mandar, with whom he maintained lifelong relations of esteem, was an active author and a close friend of Jean-Jacques Rousseau.

After his graduation, Bonald entered the Musketeers, around the end of 1773, where he remained until the suppression of that corps in 1776. Returning to Millau, he married and devoted himself to his family. Though content to devote himself to domestic life, he was soon pressured by the local *intendant* into accepting the mayoralty of Millau—an office that in practice could be compelled on aristocrats. Despite his initial reluctance to tear himself from family activities to accomplish his duties, he distinguished himself in this post.

Soon after the outbreak of the Revolution, he was elected president of his newly created department, a post he resigned upon the promulgation of the Civil Constitution of the Clergy, which placed the Catholic Church in France under the control of the secular government. As the revolutionary storm worsened, he emigrated to Heidelberg with two of his young sons, so avoiding imprisonment and probable execution under the Reign of Terror.

In Heidelberg, friendless, penniless, almost without books to refer to, and preoccupied with the education of his young sons, he composed his first work, *Théorie du pouvoir politique et religieux* ("A Theory of Power Political and Religious," 1796), a lengthy treatise in which he attempted to counter the doctrines of Rousseau and Montesquieu which, in his view, had brought about the Revolution that was devouring society in France. Although ungainly in form and at times laborious in style, this work laid down the basic principles of social analysis that would reappear with more economy and grace in his subsequent works.

As the worst frenzies of the Terror cooled in 1797, Bonald and his sons slipped across the border from Switzerland on foot, traveling across the mountains at night to avoid French border patrols. After a two-week reunion with his wife and surviving children in Montpellier—his mother and one of his daughters had died in his absence—he was obliged to go into hiding, as the persecution of aristocrats was being renewed. Bonald set out for Paris, thinking it would be easier to vanish among its crowds, and lived there incognito for two years.

The enforced isolation and inactivity of this time led to the most productive period of his intellectual life. Three major works flowed in succession from his pen. The first of these, *Essai analytique sur les lois naturelles de l'ordre social* ("Analytical Essay on the Natural Laws of the Social Order," 1800), is essentially a more economical statement of *A Theory of Power.* Next to appear was the subject of the present translation, *Du divorce,* ("On Divorce," 1801), which links a theory of the family to a theory of politics as inseparable components of a viable theory of society. This was followed by *Législation primitive* ("The First Laws," 1802), a distillation of the ideas of *A Theory of Power* into a rigorous philosophical form.

As Napoleon gradually restored order to a France shaken by the confusion and excesses of the Revolution, these writings brought Bonald increasingly into the public eye. The admirers of Bonald's works included Napoleon, who offered to reprint *A Theory of Power,* although Bonald, faithful to the royal line, resisted the Emperor's offers of patronage.

With the Restoration of the monarchy in 1814, Bonald threw himself fully into public life, and emerged as one of the principal statesmen of the regime whose restoration his works had predicted.

It fell to the new government either to confirm or to roll back the vast changes the Revolution had produced. One such change was the institution of divorce, which had been decreed in 1792 at the height of the Revolution. When the question of divorce was raised in 1815, Bonald assumed the burden of abolishing it altogether. As the leader of those opposed to divorce, he gave a crucial speech in the Chamber of Deputies, which essentially summarizes the argument of *On Divorce,* and was subsequently appointed to write the report of a government commission on the subject. Thanks largely to Bonald's unstinting efforts, France abolished divorce in 1816. (It was only reinstated under the Third Republic in 1884.)

For the rest of the Restoration, Bonald remained a highly visible figure, defending the regime, serving in various official capacities, and writing articles on a wide variety of subjects. He found time to produce several major works, notably *Recherches philosophiques sur les premiers objets des connaissances morales* ("Philosophical Inquiries on the First Objects of Moral Knowledge," 1818), a work of pure philosophy, and *Démonstration philosophique du principe constitutif de la société* ("A Philosophical Demonstration of Society's Constitutive Principle," 1830), a synthesis of all his previous political works. He died in 1840 at his small estate near Millau, in the house of his ancestors.

* * *

Bonald's very prominence as a political actor has tended to veil his significance as a political philosopher. It is difficult, in the French context, to consider Bonald without evoking the parties and slogans of the Restoration era—although this may have begun to change with the extraordinary process of national healing initiated by François Furet, the Lech Walesa of French historiography. In any event, Americans at the moment may actually have an advantage in evaluating Bonald's significance for the modern world, as it is easier for them to consider Bonald's thought in terms of its intrinsic value, rather than in terms of his location on a still-extant political spectrum.

Even in the English-speaking world, though, Bonald has been so to speak over-identified with his political party, whose shifting consensus was by no means identical with his own singularly consistent principles. The usual fashion among Anglophone conservatives has been to mention Maistre and Bonald along with Burke and then—usually without having read them—to dismiss Maistre and Bonald as "Continental absolutists," in contrast to the semiliberal Burke, who is felt to be more acceptable to the liberal center of gravity. It is certainly true that Bonald was an absolutist; but his thought covers crucial areas that are not even mentioned, let alone adequately treated, by Burke, and is even more of a departure in terms of its method.

It was the great contribution of Burke to show that the reasons for traditional institutions are necessarily unknown—an idea echoed by both Maistre and Bonald.[3] It was the great

[3] See, for instance, Maistre's *Essai sur le principe générateur des constitutions politiques* (1814), XII, and Bonald's *On Divorce*, pp. 26–27.

contribution of Bonald and Maistre to take the next step, and proceed to the investigation of this unknown territory. Their goal, in Maistre's words, was "to place an eternal barrier between the innovators and us."[4]

The French Revolution called into question the very bases of society, unlike the American Revolution that preceded it, which was admired by both Burke and Maistre. By demonstrating the function of tradition, Burke was able to refute the French Revolution in its principle. But grounded in tradition alone, conservatism becomes relativism, and consequently impotent. To the loud voice of the radical who, with a bullhorn in his hand and a mob at his back, demands "Why must things be the way they are?" the relativist conservative can only answer "Because that's the way they've always been." Let the radical once succeed in his aims, and the relativist conservative is entirely helpless: his radical traditionalism condemns him to accept "change" as a constant element in human life, and he no longer has any fixed place on which to stand.

Moreover—since the reasons for traditional institutions are unknown—naive, if heartfelt, replies are all the would-be conservative can give to the radical's insistent demands for change. Whatever the change contemplated, from abortion to socialism, and whether the institution to be demolished is valid or not, the conservative is reduced to saying, in effect, that something is wrong because it's wrong. This inherited morality is often right, but it is also mute.

It is in rising to this challenge that Bonald exceeds Burke and even Maistre. Confronted with a society already devastated by reform, he was forced to contemplate a task of restoration rather than merely one of conservation; and to accomplish it, he was obliged to seek explanations for the traditional institutions that Burke had deemed inexplicable, or at least unexplained. To counter the victorious reformers, in

[4] Joseph de Maistre, *Du Pape* (1820), ch. 1.

other words, he was obliged to demolish their specific arguments as well as their epistemology; and in doing so, it is arguable that he founded the modern discipline of sociology. Comte and Proudhon on the left, Lamennais and Maurras on the right, among many others, acknowledged Bonald as a fundamental influence in the nineteenth century; and whatever one may think of these writers individually, the notion of Bonald as a simple-minded "Continental absolutist" clearly cannot survive their unanimous acclaim.[5] That modern sociology has dead-ended as a science and become a mere methodology should summon us back to its source, to find the cause of its sterility. In this case the errors, I would suggest, lie more in the disciples than in the master.

To a vastly higher degree than any other early conservative thinker, Bonald studied the resonance phenomena of morality. If something is wrong morally, it must have resonance effects on the fabric of society. (Sociobiologists would reverse the direction of causation here and view morality itself as a resonance phenomenon of evolution.) By identifying and describing these effects, reason can demonstrate the necessity of morality to those who do not commence with implicit faith in it. (As is typical of Bonald, this position is fully compatible with Catholic doctrine, which acknowledges the capacity of human reason to investigate a variety of moral and theological issues.) Burkean theory predicts that traditional institutions will reflect sound principles; Bonald attempts to identify what those principles are. As the modern world is increasingly reformed, Burke's conservative approach is less and less ade-

[5] Bonald's other declared admirers included, among others, Napoleon, Fontanes, La Harpe, Lamartine, Sainte-Beuve, Jules Simon, and Balzac. In recent times, Robert Nisbet has explored the influence on modern sociology of French Restoration conservatives, particularly Bonald. See, for instance, *A History of Sociological Analysis,* edited by Tom Bottomore and Robert Nisbet (New York: Basic Books, 1978), pp. 80–117. See also Robert Spaemann, *Der Ursprung der Soziologie aus dem Geist der Restauration: Studien über L. G. A. de Bonald* (Munich: Kösel-Verlag, 1959).

quate, and Bonald's investigative and restorative approach is more and more necessary.

It is the peculiar insanity of our time to view every social question that arises as a disconnected element, divorced from its place in the larger scheme of things. Divorce is seen as a "women's issue," though it effects the lives of husbands, wives, fathers, mothers, boys, girls, grandparents, and the fabric of community—and affects, too, education, crime, mental illness, addiction, ultimately the economy—nay, I must stop somewhere in this list. Single motherhood is also a "women's issue," though it has precisely the same far-reaching effects. Got a problem? Slap a solution on it. Poverty? Give people money. Teenage pregnancy? Teach children about sex. Child abuse? Police the family. Drugs? Declare war on them. Homeless people? Build apartments. Another list that could be continued indefinitely.

What is wrong with these cries for compassion, these demands for generosity, which the media transmit to us every day of our lives? That they don't work, for one thing—a proposition that cannot be adequately documented here, but is demonstrated *a priori* by the fact that, after instituting each of these measures, the people who were supposed to be helped are visibly worse off than before. On a more basic level, such acts reflect a failure to grasp the interconnectedness of human affairs, the infinite feedback loops that relentlessly frustrate the targeted plans of social reformers, as they do those of socialist economists. We must move to a more basic level, to that of philosophy, to make sense of the problems that confront us, and which our putative solutions only serve to increase.

It is precisely on this level that Bonald's thought remains so interesting today. Present at the birth of leftism and rightism alike, he grasps the fundamental issues at stake with an immediacy that would in many cases be hard to replicate. His criticism of Rousseau, in particular, is often definitive, though hitherto overlooked. For example, why do so many modern anthropologists attempt to deny that cannibalism has ever been practiced, in the face of extensive evidence to the contrary? It is because their study of primitive man is a quest for Rousseau's Noble Savage. To admit the frequent ignobility of primitive peoples would strike at the heart of their entire world-view. For if primitive man turns out to be just as wicked as civilized man, then one is forced back on the doctrine of Original Sin, or its evolutionist equivalent.

Courageous in his stands, effective in his battles, constant as a friend, loved as a father, unfailingly chaste in the very salons of Paris, and consistently honest amid all the temptations of high public office, Bonald in his thought still exhibits notions that skirt, at the very least, the bounds of moral acceptability, and presage, though they do not remotely equal, the virulent racism of the late-nineteenth-century right. In this respect, Bonald stands as an object lesson in the inadequacy of current political doctrines, refuting, in some regards at least, both liberals and conservatives: liberals, by the fatal objections he raises to their fundamental assumptions; conservatives, by the example of the vile xenophobia into which his own principles periodically lead him. One must conclude that the modern world requires a political philosophy reconciling (classical) liberalism and conservatism; and that for this purpose, Bonald contains both wheat and chaff, or, one could say, food and poison, like cassava, one of the most nutritious of plants, which must be purged of a cyanide-producing sugar before it can safely be consumed.

I will not, however, attempt the extensive task of such a reconciliation here, but will insist only that Bonald's strengths are far more illuminating than his weaknesses are glaring. Unlike Burke's, his is a viewpoint that must be winnowed before it can be used—and for that very reason it is likely to produce some very interesting results in the course of its rediscovery, as it previously did in the nineteenth century.

Burke inspires a school; Bonald will inspire schools. Nevertheless, and despite all Bonald's weaknesses and Burke's glories, it is Bonald we need most today: in his reunifying vision is the antidote for the fragmentation of the modern vision—a viewpoint that has seemed so arcane as to be hopelessly unattainable, but which once recovered seems like simple common sense.

For the modern world has things exactly backwards. In truth, there are no women's questions, no men's questions, no children's questions, no blacks' questions, no whites' questions, no labor questions, no business questions: there are only social questions, which can only be answered in terms of society as a whole. Do you wish to help any of these groups? It can only be done by strengthening the bonds of society. To attempt specifically to help any of these groups necessarily corrodes those bonds, injures vital relationships, and so hurts those it purports to help—a cruel compassion, an antisocial philanthropy, a corrosive progress. Because it has lost this insight, today's conservative movement does not have enough conservative strength to stop the march of radicalism; and in this regard, however they may view his prejudices, his monarchism, or his anticommercialism, today's conservatives, whatever they call themselves, need Bonald. In this Bonald is the master, the source, without peer.

TRANSLATOR'S NOTE

The Dating of the Work

On Divorce was originally published in 1801 by Adrien Le Clère, a Paris publisher, as *Du divorce, considéré au XIXᵉ siècle relativement à l'état domestique et à l'état publique de société, par L. G. A. B. . . . .* ("On Divorce, Considered in the Nineteenth Century in Relation to the Domestic and Public States of Society, by L. G. A. B. . . . .").

The writing of *On Divorce* can be dated with some precision. The proposed Civil Code to which Bonald refers in the work was formally presented by a commission of the Council of State on 24 Thermidor, Year VIII (August 12, 1800) and published in the Year IX (September 23, 1800-September 22, 1801). Since *On Divorce* was published in 1801, and references to the proposed Civil Code occur throughout the work and are integral to the text, it is likely that Bonald began writing *On Divorce* in the fall of 1800 at the earliest.

Other evidence makes it possible to confirm and refine this dating. Years later, Bonald wrote: "It was at the request of M. Portalis senior that the author wrote *On Divorce Considered in the Nineteenth Century.*"[1] Jean-Etienne-Marie Portalis, a noted jurist, was proscribed in 1797 and only returned from exile in Germany in 1800. This would confirm that *On Divorce* was written in 1800 at the earliest. Portalis was appointed to the Council of State in 1801 and subsequently took

---

[1] Louis de Bonald, "Sur les enfants trouvés," published with "De la loi sur l'organisation des corps administratifs" (Paris: Le Clère, 1829), 86n. Bonald refers to Portalis in *On Divorce* at the end of Chapter One.

part in the writing of the Civil Code. This makes it likely that the entire work was written in 1801, after Portalis began to concern himself with the Civil Code.

The "Summation" that concludes the work was originally published as a separate pamphlet, *Résumé sur la question du divorce* (Paris: Le Clère, 1801). Unlike *On Divorce,* it shows the influence of Jacques de Maleville's pamphlet *On Divorce and Separation* (Year X [1801]), which Bonald must have read in the meantime (on Maleville, see "Summation," note 3). Since the Year X began on September 23, 1801, and the Summation was published in 1801, this dates the writing of the Summation to the fall of 1801.

Variants between Editions

For the second edition of *On Divorce* in 1805, Chapter One was heavily rewritten and somewhat expanded. The rest of the work was lightly but extensively retouched. An interesting detail is that the imperfect tense ending -ait was changed to the pre-Revolutionary spelling -oit throughout the work. The Addendum that follows the Appendix was added at this time, along with the concluding "Summation," which had already been published separately in 1801. In other respects, the work was unchanged from the first edition: in particular, only very minor edits were made to the Introduction and Conclusion.

With the second edition, Bonald evidently felt the work had assumed its definitive form, and the subsequent editions—of 1818, 1839, and 1847 (in the second edition of Bonald's *Oeuvres*)—simply reprint the second edition, with insignificant typographical variants. The 1864 text of *On Divorce* in the third edition of Bonald's *Oeuvres,* published by the abbé Migne, is more ambitious, though not always reliable. Migne provided modernized Latin spellings, which I have followed, and introduced a number of notes, which I have not, on the ground that they alter the character of the work. It is with some reluctance that I have introduced any notes at all. Most of these fall into two categories: (1) translation of Latin citations; (2) identification of French and Latin works cited.

This translation is based on the third (1818) edition of *Du divorce,* checked against the other editions. In one or two cases, I have followed readings from the first edition when these are clearer.

About the Translation

I wanted to achieve a translation that would be accessible to the general reader, without artificially modernizing Bonald's language, and which would be sufficiently rigorous to serve as a basis for intensive study by the political philosopher, without the need to refer frequently, if at all, to the original French text. For both reasons, I have rigorously used the same expressions to translate words that carry a special significance in Bonald's thought, such as *power, minister, subject, morals,* and *relationship,* as well as such recurrent expressions as *conjugal tie, marital power,* and *the faculty of divorce.* Thus French *pouvoir* is always *power,* but *puissance* is always *might.* (French *sensible* is rendered as *sensible,* which always carries its pre-twentieth-century English meaning of "sensitive, sensate, capable of being sensed.") I believe this is a translation the reader can approach with confidence, and that, unlike some works one can think of, the experience of reading this work in English is nearly indistinguishable from that of reading it in French.

Of course, if the deconstructionists are right, I may have translated Shakespeare by accident. On the other hand, if they are right, there would be as little point in translating Bonald as there is in translating Jacques Derrida.

Acknowledgments

I would like to express my appreciation to E. Christian Kopff of the University of Colorado at Boulder for his assistance in translating the Latin citations. Stephen Stertz also provided helpful advice in this area. The McCaffreys, of Conservative Book Club fame, have been unstinting in their support for this project. Robert Nisbet, Thomas Molnar, and Peter Viereck have most kindly encouraged the effort. It is a pleasure to express my debts to the eminent Russell Kirk for including this work in the Library of Conservative Thought published by Transaction and to Transaction's fearless publisher, Irving Louis Horowitz, a worthy successor to Adrien Le Clère.

Nicholas Davidson

New York
May, 1991

ON DIVORCE,

Considered in the Nineteenth Century,

in Relation to

the Domestic and Public States

of Society

If the legislator, mistaking his object, establishes a principle different from that which arises from the nature of things, the State will not cease to be agitated until it is destroyed or changed, and invincible nature has resumed her sway.

Social Contract

INTRODUCTION

IT is a fertile source of error, when treating a question relative to society, to consider it by itself, with no *relationship* to other questions, because society itself is only a group of *relationships.* In the social body as in every organized body—that is to say, one in which the parts are arranged in certain *relationships* to each other relative to a given end—the cessation of vital functions does not come from the annihilation of the parts, but from their displacement and the disturbance of their *relationships.*

How, indeed, can one treat divorce, which disunites the father, mother, and child, without speaking of society, which unites them? How can one treat society's domestic state, or the family, without considering its public or political state, which intervenes at the family's formation in order to guarantee its stability and ensure its effects? But the reason for domestic power, which unites men in the family, the reason for public power, which unites families in State bodies, lies at bottom neither in man nor in the family; for man by himself is independent of every other man, and the family of every other family. It is therefore necessary to return to the universal supreme power over all beings; that is, to the knowledge of a being superior to man, existing before human society, whose will, conservative of created beings, manifests itself in a given order of *relationships,* which, expressed by laws, constitute human power, and therefore society; to the universal power of God over man, and the duties of man toward God, which together explain the inexplicable power of man over man, and the duties which flow from it; to divine power, the knowledge and worship of which are the object of *religion* or the society which unites, which binds, from *religare*,[1] because it is the bond and reason for the other societies.

So runs the course of reason, but not that of modern philosophy; and since the question with which we are concerned, the first and most fundamental of all social questions, is the battleground on which this philosophy has been striving for so long against reason, the reader will allow me to set forth here, in some detail, the subject of their quarrel and its effects on society.

A developed reason comprehends all beings, and their existing and even possible relationships, under these three general ideas, the most general the mind can conceive: *cause, means,* and *effect,** whose perception is the basis for all judgment, and whose external reality is the foundation for all social order. To apply this principle, a little abstract perhaps, to society, reason sees in God who *wills* the first *cause;* in the *man,* whoever he may be, who *acts* to execute this will, the secondary cause, or the *means,* the *minister,* the *mediator;* and the *effect* in that order of things called *society,* which results from God's will and man's action.

Thus the supreme power lies in the supreme intelligence or God; the subordinate power lies in the subordinate intelligence or a man; and this *human being,* a *power* himself, in society's domestic order as in its public order, has *ministers* and *subjects* under him; so that the particular order, constituted like the general one, is a chain of primary *causes,* of *means* or secondary causes, and of *effects*—an order which is believable by man's reason, because he exists, and is even *sensible* in his particular action.

Ancient philosophy admitted these fundamental principles

*See the *First Laws* by the same author, in which these ideas are developed and applied to society.[2]
[1] Latin: "to bind or fasten." Author's notes are indicated by an asterisk, translator's notes by a number.
[2] Louis de Bonald, *Législation primitive* (Paris: Le Clère, 1802).

of all order and judgment; but, weak pedagogue of childish peoples, it distorted the truth with its bizarre imaginings. It sang, in its charming poetry, chaos and time, man given life by a ray stolen from Divinity, the gods speaking with men, the Golden Age, men in the beginning happy and innocent; soon all evils spread over the earth by the imprudence of a woman, masterpiece of a Divinity; only the hope of a better future left to the human race; men corrupted, at war with each other; weakness without protection from strength—*tantumque haberent,* says Cicero, *quantum manu et viribus per caedem ac vulnera aut eripere aut retinere potuissent;*[3] at last some men inspired by the gods, in order to remove men from this state of ferocity and destruction, by giving laws to societies— brilliant fictions which enclose ancient truths; antique traditions which resemble half-forgotten memories.

Pagan philosophy had retained the imprint of another primitive truth. Reason told men that the will of the Supreme Being, being sovereignly enlightened, must be perfectly fixed and immutable. The ancients believed that this will was immutable, but they did not judge it to be enlightened. They even supposed that it was blind, because it was uniform, and they made of it *destiny,* which was superior to men and even to the gods; and it is true, in a sense, that God himself obeys his own will, and that, being sovereignly free, he can do nothing against his will.

Thus paganism separated will and intelligence in God, which is absurd, and personified will under the name of *destiny,* superior to intelligence itself; while Christianity distinguishes will from action in God, and makes the action *proceed* from the will, which is in conformity with reason; so that it distinguishes God who wills by his thought alone from

---

[3] "And they would possess only what they could steal or keep by strength of hand through killing and wounding." It has not been possible to find this passage in Cicero. Somewhat similar passages, however, are found in Cicero, *Republic* 1.33, 1.42, and elsewhere.

God or rather the God-man who acts externally, and *by whom everything was made*. But let us return to the subject at hand.

Modern philosophy, born in Greece from that eternally childish people, which *always sought wisdom* outside the paths of reason, began by removing God from the universe—whether, with the atheists, it denied God all will, by denying him existence itself, or whether, with the deists, it accepted the creative will but rejected the conservative action or Providence—and to explain society, it looks no higher than man; for I shall spare the reader all that it has imagined to explain the formation of the physical universe, and even of man, without recourse to an intelligent being superior to man and the universe. It has said such incredible things on this subject; it has attributed the existence of man, this masterpiece of creation, miracle himself amid so many miracles, to causes so absurd, acting by means so ridiculous, that today, better advised, it imposes silence on its adepts by itself concerning those senseless systems, which, for the honor of the age in which we have lived, must be forgotten, if possible, and above all not transmitted to posterity. *Nec postera credant secula.*[4]

Our philosophers, with the exception of Hobbes, were far from supposing that men, prior to society, were at war with each other. "Man is born good," says Jean-Jacques Rousseau. "In the state of pure nature," says M. de Montesquieu, "men would not seek to attack each other, and peace would be their first natural law."* From then on, the state of society was no longer *necessary;* it was at most merely convenient: man did not enter into society to conserve his existence, but to increase his pleasures; and with this principle, even if our sophists still admitted belief in Divinity, it was no longer necessary to have it intervene to give laws to men, because Divinity can never

*Peace is a *state,* not a *law.*
4 "May future ages not believe it."

intervene unnecessarily; and man, born good, either had no need for laws, or was sufficiently good to give laws to men.

And in effect, these same philosophers, who had dreamed after their fashion of a pretended state of pure nature prior to all society, in which men were happy and good, suddenly conjured up wise men, *men of genius,* philosophers, teachers and benefactors of peoples, who by themselves gave laws to humankind, which received them docilely; without condescending to tell us why laws were needed by men who, living without laws, already possessed happiness and virtue; by what event naturally good beings had become bad; or finally, if men had become bad, by what privilege a few of them had been preserved from the general corruption, while all the rest, though shorn of their natural goodness, had retained its docility.

Be that as it may, one could not attribute to man the power to make laws and form society without also attributing to him the power to abolish laws and dissolve society. Thus Jean-Jacques Rousseau solemnly advances that "a people always has the right to change its laws, even the best ones; for if it wishes to harm itself, who has the right to prevent it from doing so?"* Our philosophers had sensed that if man was originally independent of man, then every man who made laws had to be *sent* to make them; and once they had rejected any divine mission, it was a necessary consequence for them to have recourse to a human mission, and to seek, in an aggregation of men, the reason for the power they did not find in one man alone.

But the people itself was only a collection of men, and it was

---

*One day people will not believe that the writer who proffered this absurdity, and this one: *The man who thinks is a depraved animal,* and so many others, was held up, in the finest place in Europe, to the veneration of the most enlightened people in the universe.

men who sent men to give laws to men. Moreover, in deferring
to the reason of one man for the most important act of society,
the institution of laws, the people recognized the inadequacy
of its reason for governing itself. It thus acted only in virtue of
its mass, or the superiority of its numbers; it was mass which
sent reason: hence Jurieu, the apostle of popular sovereignty,
could only escape this inextricable difficulty by naively affirm-
ing that "the people is the only authority which does not have
to be right to validate its acts." Which prevented any objection, and ended all argument.

These legislators, *sent* by the people or, without being sent,
acting in their name, were, in Greece, men such as Solon and
Lycurgus; in Rome, various kings, decemvirs, triumvirs, and
tribunes; and in later times, Mohammed, Luther, and a thousand others. In Greece itself, veritable patrimony of legislators, sages did not wait for their mission to come to them;
they anticipated it, and wandered around the country looking
for laws to rewrite and cities to police. Legislation was not the
bitter medicine which a sick man, far from demanding, rejects
in his delirium, and only takes when the doctor constrains him
by force; but the garment made for the convenience of a man
in the bloom of health, ample above all, and leaving the greatest liberty to his movements: a comparison which M. de Montesquieu furnishes me himself, when he says that a wise
legislator must *try* the laws on the people, to see if they suit it;
and he has passed on this error, along with many others, with
the help of a fine mind and an inimitable style.

Among these popular legislators, one allowed a father to
expose his infant, another a wife to dismiss her husband; one
here required the master to hunt down his slave, one there
recommended abominable loves; in Crete, the insurrection of
the people against a magistrate was anticipated and subject to
rules; here men slaughtered each other in public games, to
amuse their peers; there artisans seated themselves in the
courts, to judge their fellow citizens; in Greece they invented

ostracism, to rid themselves of Aristides; in Rome they were content to condemn Verres to a fine, etc., etc.; and I shall spare the reader the recitation of many other laws, and above all our revolutionary laws, which are incomparable. It is not that intelligence, more or less, was lacking in these legislations, just as there is art, and even much of it, in the leaning tower one sees at Pisa, which maintains itself outside the perpendicular, but would crumble at the slightest shock.

> *Jamjam lapsura, cadentique*
> *Imminet assimilis.*[5]

But there was nothing natural in them, nothing necessary, and men merely substituted relationships of their own devising for the relationships which the Creator, father of humankind, had established among beings.

It belongs only to the sovereignly good Being to answer to himself concerning the perfection of his works, and to *see that they are very good.** With the passage of time, men recognize the imperfection and vice of their own works; and our philosophers, better placed than the ancients to judge the effect of these human institutions, struck by their insubstantiality, and above all by the disorders these institutions had introduced into societies, broke their idol with their own hands, and declared, by the voice of Jean-Jacques Rousseau, that "man is born good, and society depraves him"; and also, "everything that is not in nature has its disadvantages, and civil society more than all the rest." Indeed, this philosopher went much further, and declared that "the man who thinks is a depraved animal." This opinion, for the rest, was not a fit of irritation on the part of a misanthrope, out of sorts with others and himself. The ideas of order, reason, justice, good, and evil,

*Genesis, ch. 1.
[5] "Now [a rock above sinners in the Underworld], at the point of slipping, overhangs them as though it were falling." Virgil, *Aeneid* 6.602.

which are the basis for all legislation, are the most general
ideas the mind can conceive; and another philosopher, Condillac, teaches us that "general ideas demonstrate the limita-
tion of our minds; God has no need of them"; and elsewhere
he tells us "animals have general ideas": so that the function of
giving laws to men, considered to be the most noble exercise
of the intelligence, would only prove its weakness and inadequacy. And indeed, it will doubtless be noticed that I cite only
the masters; many other absurdities would appear, and I
would have too great an advantage, if I chose to cite the
glosses of the disciples.

Once Jean-Jacques Rousseau had advanced that *society depraves man,* consistent with his principle, he drove man from
society, and sent him back to the state of nature, which was
prior, according to him, to society, and which he located in
savage life (we shall soon see the reason for this); a new error:
as if society consisted in the walls of our houses or the limits of
our cities, and that wherever a man is born there were not a
father, a mother, a child, a language, heaven, earth, God, and
society.

But if man was depraved by society, then he was good before
entering society. The savage state, which precedes our state of
society, was therefore a good state; so that our modern philosophers, and especially the one of Geneva, concurred with
the sentiment of those philosophers of whom Leibniz speaks,
"who see nature where there is the least art, not recognizing
that perfection always includes art." For Leibniz, instead of
locating the natural state in the original or native state, like
those philosophers, only locates it in the subsequent and
perfected state.

Once it was agreed that savage life is man's natural state, one
went into ecstasy over the industriousness of these men who,
head in hands, spend entire days without speaking a word,
crouched naked in smoke-filled cabins which they enter on all
fours; over the virtues of these men, intemperate to the point

of madness, gamblers to the point of frenzy, violent in their quarrels, vain about their looks, thieves, idlers, who make their prisoners linger through atrocious tortures, and cook and eat them; over the strength of these men who a handful of civilized men drives before it as the wind blows dust. Having begun by admiring these savages, there was little delay in imitating their ways. Men sought to return themselves to this state of pure nature, not in physical habits, too dear to softness to attempt their reformation, but in moral habits, inconvenient to the passions; and they went further than the savages themselves.

Thus the savage transmits to his children, at least by the example of his superstitions, some crude idea of invisible beings superior to men; but Jean-Jacques Rousseau forbids one to speak to a child of God and his soul before he is fifteen years old; and still he feared to give him this knowledge too early: "for who knows," he says, "if eighteen is not still too soon?" But at the same time, he neglected nothing to fortify the body with everything he took from the spirit; and thanks to his lessons, a child, even one destined by circumstances to command other men through the authority of the laws in public employments, knew how to run, jump, and swim, even knew a little geometry and natural history, pasted up plants, pinned up butterflies, classified insects, and knew nothing about the first of all sciences, the science of society's *power* and man's *duties.*

Struebat jam fortuna in diversa parte terrarum initia causasque imperii;[6] so Tacitus begins the story of one of the revolutions of the Roman empire; and one could also say, concerning the era in which these guilty doctrines began to be spread, that "philosophy was already preparing, in regions foreign to all order and society, the origins of the horrifying

---

[6] "Fortune was already preparing, in a distant part of the world, the origin and rise of a new dynasty." Tacitus, *Histories* 2.1.1.

dominion which it wielded for a time over France." Then began in Europe that revolution from which France is having so much difficulty extricating herself; and there sprang up, for the times which were to come, a race of *giants* in malice, whose uncultivated or badly cultivated minds were open to all errors, and whose hardened bodies were ready for all trials.

We have spoken of the state of nature, but we have not yet developed the larger sense which the sophists attach to this expression.

That infinite force which involves man and his systems, the peoples and their institutions, the universe itself and its vicissitudes, in a general order which particular disorders are unable to disturb, has never ceased, from the beginning of time, to inform man that he is not the cause of society, but only a means within it, and most often only an instrument. Forced to recognize a will in the world superior to his will, and an action stronger than his action, the ancient philosopher had called it *destiny;* the modern philosopher called it *nature,* an occult, blind, unyielding force; and as the ancients had explained everything by the immutable decrees of destiny, the moderns did so by the forces of *nature* and the laws of *nature*. This nature was for them at once the *cause, means,* and *effect;* creative and created, ordering and ordered, simultaneously active and passive; and such was the prodigious weakening of human thought that some sought to expound these absurdities, and others believed they understood them.

The modern philosophers were much less excusable in their errors than the pagan philosophers had been. The latter, placed closer to the origin of things, had neither a large enough number of observations, nor reliable enough means of collecting them, to acquire a clear idea of the order which societies obey even in their revolutions, as the stars do in theirs; whereas the modern sages, coming at the end of time, enriched by all the observations which history has handed down to us, and which the art of printing has conserved, could, by comparing ancient and modern times, pagan and Christian societies—the weakness, ignorance, and vices of some, the strength, enlightenment, and virtues of others—judge principles by their results, and conclude that there is, in Christian societies, a continuously operating principle of perfection and strength, other than that nature, blind and devoid of intelligence, whose action could not be explained without falling into pitiful contradictions.

Nevertheless Jean-Jacques Rousseau, who, from the religious opinions of his childhood, had retained belief in a God and some notion of divine revelation, sought to reconcile the former and the latter with the system of nature then in vogue, and above all with the hatred of all visible authority, whose principle he had acquired from the dogmas of the pretended Reformation. He admitted God as a cause, but rejected the intervention and ministry of *any human being,* and he says, "What God wills man to do, he does not tell him through another man, he tells it to him himself, and writes it at the bottom of his heart." But he only displaced the problem; for if man is *obliged* to read the laws, to understand and follow them, then there is no more free will in man, no more good, no more evil, no more just, no more unjust, no more laws, no more society, and man is a stone which gravitates toward a center. If on the contrary man can neglect to read his own heart, err in the reading, or disobey after having read, then there must be an authority which makes him attentive or docile to these laws, and an authority which interprets them; and from whence shall man acquire the mission to interpret, for man, laws written by God himself at the bottom of his heart, or to force him to follow them? But this writing could not be material; it was therefore intellectual, and so, in whatever manner one understands him, Jean-Jacques Rousseau entered fully into the system of *innate ideas,* which the philosophers had so ridiculed; and the school had never supported them in a more rigorous sense.

The dominant party among modern sophists did not concur with the *theist* opinions of Jean-Jacques Rousseau, or with the origin, confused as it was, which he gave to natural laws; and that philosopher himself never ceased to attribute his real and imagined miseries to the hatred borne him by the atheists. But man, body as well as spirit, cannot be governed by pure abstractions devoid of all reality: the apostles of *naturalism* were obliged, in order to make themselves understood, to realize their abstract term *nature*, as they had realized the abstract term *people*; and as they had seen the whole people in the *sages* who gave it laws, so they saw nature, and all of nature, in sensible and material beings. One should note that all religious worship is itself merely the *realization* of the abstract idea of God, who, without this *reality*, would soon be erased from thought. Thus paganism depicted its gods as *present and real*, in its many representations . . . ; thus Christianity depicts Divinity *really present*. . . . But let us continue.

Animals, rocks, plants, all the bodies which exist in space, and those bodies alone, were thus *nature*; and the order of laws, invariable within each kind and constant for all kinds, to which bodies are subject for their reproduction and conservation, was also nature. In the natural laws of the physical order, and especially in the laws of the animal *kingdom*, one sought the reason for even the social functions of man; and so was seen the introduction of the most crude and abject kind of materialism, the system of *animalism*, which distinguishes the present era, and was the application and result of the system of abstract *naturalism* of Baron d'Holbach and his school.*
Then, if I dare say it, *night fell* in society; the murkiest systems on God, on man, on society, on *power*, and on *duty* appeared; all intelligence was obscured: *Animalis homo non percipit ea*

---

*This is the school which gave rise to the *System of Nature*.[7]
[7] Paul-Henri-Dietrich Thyry, baron d'Holbach, *Système de la nature* (London, 1770).

quae sunt spiritus; stultitia enim est illi, et non potest intelligere.*8

Man, a *reasonable animal,* was defined by first considering his physical qualities and the animal functions he shares with the beasts. It is roughly thus that the negro calls the orangutan *a man who does not speak.* Philosophy stopped halfway through these definitions; it made an animal of man, and a man of the monkey, and it does not despair that one day the monkey will learn to reason. It has gone even further in its terms, and defined man as "an organized and sensible *mass* which receives spirit from everything in its environment and from its needs";† a definition which, in the system of the *animalists,* could be applied in its entirety to a dog, which is also, according to them, *an organized and sensible mass which receives spirit* from the man who trains it *and from its needs.*

Man, considered by a true philosophy,‡ is *an intelligence served by organs;* the beasts, on the contrary, are *organs moved by an instinct;* and these two definitions express the beings to which they refer by the characteristic and essential traits of their respective natures: man, by the will which directs his actions; the beast, by the necessity which determines

*Saint Paul, 1 Corinthians 2.14.
†This definition is by M. de Saint-Lambert, from his *Catechism of Philosophical Morality,* in five volumes, which is as riddled with errors as his *Poem of the Seasons* is gracious and brilliant.9
‡*Anima per se,* says Stahl, *nihil agere potest et sine corporeorum organorum ministerio. . . . Anima per sensoria organa active excubias agit.*10
8 "The man of this life does not perceive the things of the spirit; to him they are foolishness and he cannot understand them."
9 *Le catéchisme universel,* in vol. 2 (Year V [1797]) of Jean-François, marquis de Saint-Lambert, *Oeuvres philosophiques,* 5 vols. (Paris: Agasse, Years V-IX [1797–1801]; a sixth, undated volume was subsequently added). The *Catéchisme universel* was almost immediately republished in Saint-Lambert's *Principes des moeurs,* 6 vols. (Paris: Agasse, Year VI [1798]), vol. 2. By the same author, *Les saisons, poème* (Paris: P. Didot l'aîné, 1769).
10 "The soul can do nothing by itself without the help of the bodily organs. . . . The soul actively keeps its watch through the sense organs."

its movements. And what comparison, indeed, can be established between the being which makes all other beings, and
even the animals, serve as ministers of his will and instruments
of his action, and beings which are obeyed by no other being,
because they are not understood by it, and which act without
instruments or means, without intermediary, upon the beings
necessary to their conservation? For that is the essential difference between man and beast. Man never *acts* without a
means or *mediator* between his will and the action resulting
from it, because man grasps the relationship between himself
and the means he uses, and between the means he uses and
the effect he wishes to obtain. Thus man conceives of the
relationship between himself and the cart he causes to move;
the relationship between the different parts of the cart; the
relationship between himself and the horses he guides, and
between the horses and the cart they draw; finally, the relationship between this whole device and the earth he cultivates,
and the grain which comes from it, etc., etc.; and it is precisely in this perception of relationships that intelligence consists. The beast, on the contrary, either uses no *means,* or if it
does, like the nest which birds make for their eggs, then the
invariable uniformity of this little structure in each species
sufficiently demonstrates that it is not designed by an intelligence proper to each individual. The beast thus conceives of
no relationships; thus it has no intelligence. Does the wiliest
cat ever think of closing the hole by which the mouse has
escaped from it a hundred times? Has the beaver, eternally
captured by the hunter at the mouth of its aquatic cabin, ever
varied its construction? Man, on the contrary, ceaselessly
discovers new relationships, imagines and uses new means,
and extends and perfects his action by them; and today a weak
child can, by pressing a trigger, slaughter those colossal animals whose sight confounds us, or, by touching an ember to a
trail of powder, make a mountain burst into pieces, or annihilate a vast edifice in the blink of an eye. Happy would man be if

he used his industry only for his well-being and the progress of society.

Our philosophers, forced to recognize this marvelous capacity for industry, did not attribute it to man's intelligence but to his organs. They attributed the admirable order which reigned in this house to the lackeys' service rather than the master's wisdom. In the form of man's hand, Helvétius discovered the reason for the difference he could not help noticing between man's actions and the beast's movements. He failed to notice that man is not intelligent because he is industrious, but industrious because he is intelligent; and that he is not, as Aristotle says, superior to the animals because he has a hand, but that he has a hand because he is superior to the animals (*De part. anim.* 3.10); that his industry is the daughter of his intelligence, as his action is the daughter of his will; and that man's hand, as admirable as its form is, if denuded of the instruments supplied by intelligence is at bottom less deft, and above all less strong, than the elephant's trunk.

And observe that at the same time Helvétius was locating all our intelligence in the structure of our hand, Condillac was locating all our acquired knowledge, or virtually so, in the perfection of our sense of touch, which he made, no one knows why, the sense which regulates all the others.

Be that as it may, man was no longer anything but a somewhat better formed animal. Some gave beast and man only senses and sensations, others gave them an intelligence of the same kind. Even the various degrees of intelligence in the different animals, including man, were measured by the different degrees of acuity of the *facial angle,* happy invention of our modern physiologists; and it was not seen that there is intelligence in even the dullest of men who brings together two pieces of wood to make a fire, and no intelligence in the well-trained dog that seeks at the bottom of the water for the stone which I have thrown, which I myself no longer recognize, and that, sensible to the vagaries of temperature, does not know, by itself, how to find any external means to protect itself from them.

Thus one must observe that those philosophers, such as Descartes and his disciples, who attribute the most to human intelligence, including even innate ideas, make the beasts into pure machines; while those, like Condillac and others, who attribute intelligence, including even general ideas, to the beasts, deny the most to human intelligence, make it depend entirely on the senses, and make, or virtually so, *man* a *machine* or a *statue:* a total divergence of opinion, which perfectly characterizes the century of mind and the century of matter.

The same philosophers who, in certain physical resemblances between man and the animals, had sought the reason for our individual habits, thought they would find the reason for our social functions there as well.

They noted that the beasts were only moved by the sensation of pain and the appetite for pleasure, and they immediately established in principle that man could only be motivated by his personal interest, which they made to consist in seeking pleasure and avoiding pain.

With a little reflection, though, they would have observed that, in the brief moments of its life during which it has an end relative to its peers, like the female and sometimes the male at the times of incubation and nursing, the animal, far from being moved by the individual sensation of pain or pleasure, is motivated by another principle, and neglects even the care of its own conservation, suffering pain and often death in order to defend its young, even in the weakest and most timid species. From this one would have concluded that man, who does not devote himself to the service of other men, even that of his own children, by any involuntary instinct or unconscious movement, can only do so by a free and enlightened will; that in consequence what is for the beast a passing necessity becomes for man a habitual duty; and that if self-love determines man's will in individual actions which have no object but his own satisfaction, only the love of others can determine his will in social actions of which others are the subject. And do not subtilize to the point of saying that the love of others is only, in this case, self-love properly understood; for then we are only arguing about words, as David Hume observes; and I would demand that one explain to me what personal interest man can find in devoting himself to the service of others in positions which are obscure, unrewarded, and dangerous, if one supposes that his devotion contains no motive founded in the love of others; a sacrifice of self to others, which only a being superior to man can command of him, because only such a being can inspire him with the necessary strength and confer on him the prize.

This disposition to see in man nothing but an animal determined by animal laws has led our philosophers to recognize no duties but in the fulfillment of animal laws, and no virtue but in the fulfillment of those duties. Allow me to explain.

Man, like the beast, has received the faculty of reproducing himself in a being similar to himself; but this faculty, *necessitated* in the beast, and at a given moment, is purely voluntary in man. The sophists pretended it was *necessary* in man, and there was no further question but of involuntary needs and irresistible attractions, inspiring many bad novels and even more bad philosophy. When the union of the sexes became a duty, the sublime wish to consecrate oneself whole and undistracted to the service of others, and to know no family but public society—this vow of celibacy which is practiced, without uttering it, by the flower of a nation's youth which the service of society keeps under arms—was no longer seen as anything but a crime of *lèse-nature,* an outrage to its laws, an offense, finally, against God, against man, and against society.

Woman, like the female of the animals, has the faculty of nursing her infant; but this faculty, necessitated in the animal, which cannot replace itself with others, is purely voluntary in woman; and this duty, for it can be such, is subject to a host of circumstances which can modify its obligation. Jean-Jacques Rousseau put the trumpet to his lips, and one would have thought that before him all women were unnatural mothers and all children unhappy orphans. In the fervor of his philosophic zeal, this so very *sensible* man neglected to examine whether the moral causes which develop sensibility in man, and which do not exist in the animal, could not corrupt a mother's milk, particularly in those conditions where man, less preoccupied with domestic tasks than with public cares, and less with needs than with sentiments, more exposed to the sorrows of life because he tastes more of its comforts, has a heart less resistant to painful affections, and a soul more open to the passions' deadly impressions; and Jean-Jacques Rousseau, *in the name of nature,* made it a duty for all mothers to nurse their children themselves, like the females of the animals, and for the same reason. Perhaps he even thought that he had caught out religion, which, contenting itself to inspire women with moderate desires and forbid them all alien affections, by the duty which it enjoins on them of a modest and busy life, places them naturally in a situation where the nursing of their children is without conflict for themselves or danger to their children, and which perhaps, carrying our views further, fears, under certain circumstances, anything which could serve young spouses as a cause or pretext for living apart, even momentarily. It is true that Jean-Jacques Rousseau speaks, and even eloquently so, of domestic duties, and declaims against the arts, and even, for he attacks everything, against the sciences; but at the same time—such is the disorder of ideas which religion does not direct—he wrote operas and novels, and of all novels, the one which has most misled women's imaginations and corrupted their hearts. In any event, by hearing nursing described as a duty, women made it into a fashion conducive to beauty, as it had been in the declamations of the sophist; and softened or impassioned mothers, who, in sacrificing to fashion, wished to give up none of their pleasures, nor even any of their disorders, transmitted to their children, along with their milk, their exhaustion or the bitterness of their blood, and prepared them a premature death or a languishing life. Useful and respected races were extinguished or enfeebled. Many mothers perished as victims of their taste for novelty, far more than from their duties, and more than one woman, forced to contain her anguish, poisoned her son because she had lost her lover.

The disadvantage of this confusion of ideas and duties is perceptible. Obligations are owed to the physical being only in consideration of the moral being; and the duty of nursing can be replaced for man, even by the animal. But the duties owed to the moral being, those duties of which philosophy may well speak in its ostentatious declamations, but for which religion alone inspires the will and gives the courage, are absolute duties, independent of times, places, and men, and duties from which nothing can dispense us. Now, philosophy was weakening the respect for religion every day; and the women whom it infatuated with its doctrine, proud to accomplish the easy duty of giving the breast to a *well-turned* child, were far from devoting themselves to the obscure and trying task of sacrificing their time to its instruction, and their tastes to the good example they owed it.

Fathers and mothers, considered by philosophy as males and females, considered their children as merely their young. Affections no longer directed by reason, and a soft and undignified domestic education, took the place of those relations of authority and submission between parents and children whose last traces the generation that is ending witnessed in its youth. Children who had ideas of equality with their parents in their minds, and sentiments of insubordination to their wishes in their hearts, allowed themselves, in speaking to them, the *tutoiement,* which in the French language, addressed to a man, expresses familiarity or contempt; and parents, conscious of their weakness, not daring to be the masters, aspired to be their children's *friends, confidants,* and too often accomplices. There were still fathers, mothers, and children in France; but there was no longer a *power* in the family, no longer a *minister,* no longer a *subject,* no longer a domestic society; and political society was shaken to its very foundations.

Everything became feeble in human affections, and grief most of all. Men who saw each other through the senses alone believed that all was lost when they ceased to see. Grief became immoderate, and consequently ostentatious and short-lived: more than one widowhood began with resolutions of suicide only to end, even too quickly, with a second marriage. A sort of pagan grief, attaching itself to the vain remains of a loved one, replaced those griefs among Christians which, although profound, were filled with a consolation of immortality, which religion maintains, even by its practices. People played with death, so to speak; it was worn like a necklace and bracelets; it was clothing, it was furniture;* and sometimes a spouse, in his hypocritical grief, would embalm the heart he had deeply injured.

This universal materialism, this disposition to see all things in man and society in terms of the senses, passed from domestic society into public society, where it worked the same ravages.

If man only lived by a physical existence, then he lost everything, absolutely everything, by being deprived of it; physical death was a misfortune beyond recompense, and far from being a cure for any evil, it was itself the greatest of evils. Human justice therefore did not have the right to condemn a man to death, even the murderer and the parricide, or to remedy an evil by an equally great evil; and philosophy every-

---

*We have seen a proposal to make utensils of glass or porcelain from the ashes of one's parents; and just a few years ago, a police ordinance permitted a mother to burn the body of her daughter and collect the ashes, in the manner of the pagans.

where proposed, and in some States effected, the abolition of the death penalty, society's first means of conservation. Not only could public authority not inflict the death penalty on the citizens, but it had above all to embellish their lives; and one saw the governments, as though carried away by a sudden mania for *philanthropy*—for that is the consecrated word—dreaming of nothing but money for themselves and commerce for their subjects; placing virtue in the taste for the arts, strength in population, wealth in specie, happiness in pleasure; neglecting public instruction, and above all the instruction of example; destroying religious establishments in order to establish factories and theaters, and believing they had fulfilled all their duties to their peoples by giving them *bread and circuses.*

The taste for purely domestic pleasures won out over the honor of exercising public functions. Thanks to these abject doctrines, the civil and military officers, the ministers of religion and the State, the heads of State themselves, *regarded themselves as abuses,* whose reformation they both expected and provoked. Everyone wanted to be on his own lands, with his own books, with his own friends, occupied with his own business, and even more so with his own pleasures. Public life was nothing but an enslavement; one *took pleasure* only in private life. The State was no longer seen as anything but a mine to exploit; it was no longer on the strength of honor, but on the strength of money, that it could make itself served; like those despised masters who can only find servants by offering higher wages.

The sciences which are called *natural,* and which would be much better named *material,* because their subject is the relationships between bodies, took precedence over the social and intellectual sciences—theology, ethics, politics, and jurisprudence—which treat the relationships between intelligent beings; and by the same token, the mechanical arts, the arts of physical man, were cultivated with greater taste and success than the arts of the mind, eloquence and poetry, the noblest expression of the thinking being. Our great poets of the last century, and those of our own century who still belong to that memorable era of the human mind, had walked in the light which deep thinkers, their contemporaries, had spread on the natures of God and man, and on their relationships; and with an inimitable perfection they had expressed man, his duties, his virtues, and his passions. In our century, in which a dismal *ideology*—which is only a chapter in the science of man—has been substituted for the lofty and intellectual metaphysics of Plato, Saint Augustine, Descartes, Malebranche, Fénelon, and Leibniz, and has identified all our ideas with our sensations, and in which the physical sciences have almost exclusively been cultivated, poetry has taken on the same character. It has succeeded in depicting the senses and matter; the bantering, voluptuous and even obscene, or *georgic* and descriptive genre has won out over the lyrical and dramatic one; and in this regard, Voltaire in his well-known poem, Bernard, Dorat, Roucher, Saint-Lambert, and Delille are sons of their century, as Corneille, the two Racines, and Jean-Baptiste Rousseau were sons of theirs.

To this same principle must be attributed the noticeable tendency, in the literary works of our time, to descend from the imitation of noble and public nature to the imitation of domestic and familiar nature. Heroic tragedy, high comedy, and grand opera began in France under Louis XIV; drama, which is a sort of bourgeois tragedy, vaudeville, and comic opera are inventions of our time; and already we have seen comedy, no longer attacking absurdities or vices, but people themselves, returning to the satyrical license of the plays of Aristophanes. In the visual arts, the same character appears: the architecture of the century of Louis XIV was more concerned with exterior decoration, that of our century with interior and domestic arrangements; the rustic and crude nature of English gardens has replaced the magnificent symmetry of the designs of *Le Nôtre;* the school of Le Brun painted the public man engaged in religious or political actions; the modern school paints the domestic man, even in a savage or naked state; and in all, an extreme facility of morals, so dangerous to an advanced people, has expelled the austere and irksome constraint of the morals of our fathers. It is above all in novels, which necessarily express the time in which they are written, that one sees the difference between the two periods. At one time they contained great characters and worthy sentiments; in ours, obscure characters and petty passions. The former speak of tenderness to be sacrificed to duty, the latter of pleasures to be preferred to all else; the former recount enterprises and adventures, the latter, intrigues; and even when they speak of love alone, in the former, it is to win the heart of a lady; in the latter, it is, everything revealed, to seduce a woman; and *Clarissa* only passes, and rightly so, for the best novel of our time because it is the faithful expression of our morals;[11] for a book suffices to paint a century.

From these opinions which make man a plant in his life, an animal in his functions, there followed, as an inevitable consequence, the celebrated doctrine of the influence of climate on our customs and duties. One sought to explain everything in man and society with this influence of climate, which is combated even by modern philosophers, among others by David Hume, and refuted by reason and history.* There was no

---

*The ancient rhetoricians wrote down the *loci communes*[12] of eloquence; one could also write down the *commonplaces* of philosophy, for the use of young philosophers: the influence of climate, the prodigious antiquity of the world, the state of pure nature, the balance of powers, the benefits of commerce, etc., etc.; and then the Crusades, the expulsion of the Moors from Spain, the enterprises of the Popes, and so many other things which could make a large book that would serve marvelously to make smaller ones.

[11] Samuel Richardson, *Lettres angloises, ou Histoire de Miss Clarisse Harlove* (*sic*), translated by the abbé A.-F. Prévost, 6 vols. (London: Nourse, 1751). Subsequent French edition: *Clarisse Harlowe*, translated by M. Le Tourneur, 7 vols. (Geneva: Barde, Manget, 1785–1786). Orig. English ed.: *Clarissa, or the History of a Young Lady*, 7 vols. (London, 1748).

[12] "Commonplaces."

concern with the far stronger, and solely decisive, influence of
the political and religious institutions which modify man, and
can go so far as to change his physical constitution; and it was
not seen that the knowledge which follows civilization, born in
the Orient with religion and with man himself, had been spread
in stages, by the Jews in the ancient world, by the Christians in
the modern one, and always by the *people of God;* and that all
the great conquests which precede civilization have indiscriminately ravaged the North and South, wherever softened
peoples have offered an easy prey to simple and poor nations.

It is different thoughts which religion inspires in man, a
different character which it gives to society. Religion brings
order to man's mind, by teaching him that there is a universal
cause of universal effects or of the universe: a cause which is
essentially perfect, since it is sovereignly powerful, whereas
man is originally imperfect; and it tells us nothing but what an
enlightened reason acknowledges of God, and a deadly and
daily experience teaches us of man.

If God is good, if man is inclined to evil (for God himself
could not make the work as perfect as the workman), it is a
necessity that God has given man means to preserve himself
from the effect of his malice, and I perceive the motive for laws
and the reason for society. But when my reason clearly grasps
the *why* for the laws God has given men, my imagination,
which strays, wishes to penetrate the *how* of this transmission,
and it seeks *images* where only *ideas* are required. These
divine laws are fundamental, primitive laws, of which all
human and subsequent laws must be the more or less immediate* but always natural consequences; and the human legislator should declare or promulgate the laws, and not invent
them. This divine and natural legislation, outside of which
there is only misery for man, never develops better than where
men, delivering themselves to the march of time and the

*See the *First Laws.*

irresistible course of things, do not disturb it with their precipitate operations; and that is why, among Christian nations, the one with virtually no written political law, and no known legislator, was the strongest, most spiritual, the best, finally, and best constituted in Europe.

Religion brings order to society, because it explains the reason for power and duty to man. A head of society who knows the source of his power wields it with confidence and consequently with strength, and like God, from whom he proceeds, he knows no benevolence but justice; while the subject, sure of the reason for his duties, obeys without murmur and even with joy. But this religion which is accused of favoring tyranny, and which is the principle of all true liberty, places limits on power by placing them on duty. It teaches the heads that they cannot attempt everything, because their subjects do not owe them everything; and at the same time that it mandates *active* obedience, which political society requires from all of its ministers alike, it commands *passive* and hence insurmountable resistance whenever human power is in manifest contradiction with divine power, because then it is no longer power but passion or impotence, *impotentia;* whereas philosophy, which commands a passive obedience to its laws, or rather its orders, makes a duty of active resistance or insurrection.

Thus religion, which places God at the head of society, gives man an elevated idea of human dignity, and a profound sentiment of men's independence; and philosophy, which goes looking everywhere for men who raise themselves above their fellows in order to give them laws, always grovels at the feet of some idol: in Asia, at the feet of Mohammed; in Europe, at the feet of Luther, of Jean-Jacques Rousseau, of Voltaire; and rejecting the God of the universe, it makes gods of all men in whom it recognizes talent and rediscovers its opinions.

It is because religion essentially encloses the principles of all *order* that, when men born with great talent for government, which religion does not confer, have been animated with its spirit or accustomed to its practices, they have administered States with strength and wisdom; as witness Suger, Jiménez, Sixtus V, Richelieu; and one can even note that the strongest of them have been those who, from monastic institutions, had drawn the habit of an austere rule and a prompt obedience.

I know that philosophy opposes a philosopher-king of recent times to these great names. I do not dispute his military talent or the luster which he gave his reign; but the people he has formed have not yet passed the test of time and misfortune. Events will teach us whether the strength of a State lies in its armies or its principles, and whether, given equal abilities in the head, there is as much conservative and defensive strength in this monarchy as in certain other States in Europe.

Everything in the system of the Christian religion is natural to man's thought, because everything in it resembles his action. If man sees a supreme cause or universal power in the universe which willed everything that exists, a universal minister, means or mediator *by whom everything was made,* and universal effects *subject* to this great action called the *universe;* if he perceives general laws, and a universal, general, immutable order, punishments and rewards, he also sees himself as the cause of many effects, and as a power (domestic or public) acting through his ministers, upon his subjects and for his subjects; he sees a particular order, laws, punishments, rewards, etc. If his reason tells him that God is good, his conscience tells him that he can become so, and he finds the means, for his will, in the lessons religion gives him; for his action, in the examples it sets before his eyes; for, when great duties command the greatest sacrifices of him, and even that of life, philosophy tells him to *listen,* but religion tells him to *look. Aspice et fac secundum exemplar.*[13]

---

[13] "Look and follow the model." Exodus 25.40.

It is because the Christian religion is in conformity with the order of natural relationships between beings, and is therefore as natural to our reason as it is opposed to our penchants, that it establishes itself with ease among peoples whose education it begins, and which, still in their native ignorance, do not oppose a spirit preoccupied by error to its doctrine. These peoples enter naturally upon the road of civilization which it opens to them, and their good sense leads them to discover, between the invisible order of which they are told and the visible order whose agents they are, that perfect analogy* which is the mark of the works of an infinite intelligence, acting by an infinite power, the surest rule of our judgments, and the firmest principle of our actions; so that it is possible to say, with complete truth, that there is nothing more supernatural to man, and more natural as a whole, than religion.

Modern philosophy, on the contrary, which supposes so many effects without causes, and subjects without a power, or even in God a will without action, man naturally good, and yet giving himself laws to become so, the wife equal to the husband, the child to the father, the subject to the power, overturns order in our thoughts as in our actions, disorders man, troubles society, and produces men without reason, even when they have much intelligence, just as it produces societies without stability, even when they wield much external strength.

Thus all doctrines concerning society are divided into two diametrically opposed viewpoints.

The Christian religion teaches that man is born inclined to evil, and that he finds in society the law which rectifies his penchants.

Modern philosophy teaches that "man is born good, and society depraves him."

One, which judges our penchants to be depraved, gives us laws to combat them.

---

*Condillac is extremely hostile to proofs deduced by analogy.

The other, which judges our inclinations to be good, gives us laws to encourage them.

One, which views man as originally disordered, looks outside man for the rule of his penchants, and consequently for the motive of his duties and the reward of his virtues.

The other, which views man as originally good, does not look beyond man for the rule of his duties, a rule which it locates in his sensations;* and consequently it makes virtue a sensation of physical well-being, and vice an uneasiness, a sensation of pain; and it can neither console the good who suffer, nor restrain the wicked who prosper.†

But religion will triumph, "because order," as Malebranche says, "is the inviolable law of minds," and because beings, in the intellectual order as in the sensible one, sooner or later obey their laws. Already in Europe we see all the men of

---

*This doctrine of sensations is not of this century, and already Jurieu had said, *System,* p. 453, that "one senses truth in the divine books, as one senses light when one sees it, heat when one sits by the fire, the sweet and bitter when one eats."[14] This principle leads to every kind of fanaticism.

†Thomas Hobbes judged man to be originally bad, and he sought the motive for society in the passions of men; but he went astray when he thought he had found the cure for evil in evil itself, the reason for laws in violence, and consequently the just and unjust in men's permission or prohibition. This is what made Leibniz say, "One finds in Hobbes, and abundantly so, the deepest truths mingled with errors of the most dangerous consequence."

Luther viewed man as bad, but so bad that he even lacks the ability to become good, and is good by the grace of God alone, and without any action on his part. But if man does not have the strength to acquire, he does not have the ability to lose, and the dogma of *imputative justice* necessitated that of *inamissible justice.* Thus some wish man to be born good, and others that once good he cannot become bad. I note with pleasure that M. Kant, whose philosophy is creating such a stir in Germany, approximates the dogmas of Christianity, and recognizes "a subjection of the moral law to the principle of self-love, which is the ancient sin of man, from which follows the totality of his subsequent evil actions . . . , an evil which must be expressed under the term *original fault.*" Literary notice on M. Immanuel Kant, from the *Northern Spectator.*[15]

[14] Pierre Jurieu, *Le vrai système de l'Eglise et la véritable analyse de la Foy* (Dordrecht: Veuve de Caspar et T. Goris, 1686).

[15] *Le spectateur du Nord,* 24 vols. (pub. 1797–1802).

letters justly celebrated for their intelligence and erudition acknowledging or defending the necessity of the Christian religion, and setting the seal of its immortality upon their works; for let writers beware: all works in which the principles of order are denied or combatted will disappear from the memory of men, whatever noise they may have made among their contemporaries; and only those in which these principles are defended or respected will pass to posterity, and occasionally deserve the honor, greatest of all, to be counted among the classic books which serve to form man for society. It is a fine observation of the *Quintilian* of our century that, of all our works of literature, those most distinguished for their originality and style are, in all genres, those on which religion has placed its stamp; for since speech is the expression and image of thought, the greatest truth in ideas naturally produces the highest perfection in discourse.[16]

I shall conclude with a word on the particular subject of this work, and the reader will doubtless not judge that I have strayed from it in this introduction; for I have had to prove that religion is in conformity with reason, since in discussing the law of divorce I establish that it is only contrary to religion because it is opposed to reason.

In the course of this writing, I have reasoned on the assumption that democracy, which may be appropriate to a municipality existing under the protection of a great State, at Pontoise or in the canton of *Zug*, cannot endure in a large society. This truth is no longer disputed, even by pride, and is at most

---

[16] This is almost certainly a reference to Chateaubriand. In a characteristic expression of this idea, Chateaubriand writes: "In a word Christianity takes nothing from the poet of *natural* characters, such as antiquity was able to represent them, and offers him in addition its *influence* on these same characters. It therefore necessarily increases his *power*, since it increases his *means*, and multiplies dramatic *beauties*, by multiplying the *sources* from which they emanate." François-Auguste-René, vicomte de Chateaubriand, *Génie du Christianisme* ("The Genius of Christianity"; Paris: Gallimard, 1978; orig. ed. 1802), p. 672 (part 2, bk. 2, ch. 8).

contested only by interest. I say democracy, and I have no need to explain this expression; for the word *Republic*, which I have often used, in itself defines no particular form of government, and is synonymous with public State and political society. It is in this general sense that the best writers of the last century used it, M. Bossuet, in a thousand places, and La Fontaine, when he said,

> In the works of Mars, serving the republic.

Jean-Jacques Rousseau himself, in the *Social Contract*,[17] applies this term, and deliberately so, to all forms of government indiscriminately, and he says somewhere that "monarchy itself can be a republic."

Strongly persuaded that divorce, decreed in France, will found her misfortune and that of Europe, because France, from a thousand native and acquired circumstances, has received the power to govern Europe by her strength and enlightenment, and consequently the duty to edify it by her example; and certain that divorce came to us from the same foreign inspiration which, in the same period, dictated so many disastrous laws to France, I have been obliged to fight the proposal for it with all the means drawn from domestic and public society which my case afforded, and to set forth all the truths which could make it triumph. The truth is always useful to society, whatever sophists who see the truth in their imaginations may say, since society never perishes but from failing to know it; and that is why it may be as great a crime to keep it captive as to persecute it. But truth, which is nothing but the knowledge of the natural relationships between beings, is *generally* true, independent of times, men, and circumstances; and reason, which can only intend to be useful to society, by making truth known to men, remains, as much as possible,

---

[17] Jean-Jacques Rousseau, *Du contrat social* (Amsterdam: Mich. Rey, 1762; many subsequent editions).

among the heights of *generalities,* where absolute, essential truth is pure and unmixed like the principle from which it emanates; for it could not descend from thence without entering the *intermediate region* of particular considerations, where men's passions form the clouds which obscure it and the lightning bolts which shatter it.

I hope, then, that one will find, in this little writing on an important subject, an ardent love of truth, along with the care which truth itself enjoins to raise no obstacles to it from any motive of personal interest or vanity. Those who suffer from society should suffer only for society; a jealous mistress, she takes no account of the most extreme pains which her friends suffer for themselves alone, or of even the most glorious works if she is not their sole object; and reason itself condemns those men of whom Tacitus speaks, "who, working only for their renown, have sought an ambitious death in audacious enterprises, with no utility to the public thing"; *Qui plerique per abrupta, sed in nullum reipublicae usum, ambitiosa morte inclaruerunt.*[18]

---

[18] Tacitus, *Agricola* 42.5.

CHAPTER 1

Of the Proposed Civil Code, Presented by the Commission of the Council of State Named by the Government

WHEN the question of the dissolubility or indissolubility of the conjugal tie arose in Europe at the beginning of the sixteenth century, the heads of the Reformation and their opponents, rigid theologians all, considered it a religious question, or at least a question for religion to decide; and in the same book, and in practically the same passages, some found the toleration of the conjugal tie's dissolution, while others found the explicit law of its indissolubility.

It was a veritable civil war in the Christian world, which soon led to bloodier ones in the political world; and in which those who rose against the doctrine received in Europe believed they were respecting the dogma by attacking the discipline, rather like those political factions which struggle to gain sole control of the administration, while they all assert their loyalty to the constitution.

Different times, different spirit. The authors of the proposed Civil Code,*[1] after having taught us that "what marriage in

---

*Although this proposed code was not adopted, and another has been substituted for it since the publication of the first edition of this work, as the same principles on marriage presided over the new composition, it was not thought necessary to change anything that is said here.

[1] *Projet du code civil, présenté par la commission nommée par le Gouvernement le 24 thermidor an VIII* (Paris: Imprimerie de la République, Year IX [1801]). This was the draft version of France's *Code civil*. After extensive

itself is was previously unknown, and it is only in recent times that men have acquired precise ideas on marriage . . . ," have become convinced that "marriage as it existed before the establishment of Christianity, which preceded all positive law, and which derives from the very constitution of our being, is neither a civil nor a religious act, but a natural one, which attracted the attention of the legislator, and which religion has consecrated." (*Introduction to the proposed Civil Code.*)

It is all the more useful to discuss the principles advanced in the passage just cited in that they have provided the basis for all the laws proposed on the faculty of divorce, from the first such proposal to that which received the legislator's sanction.

How could one maintain in France, after fifteen centuries of public profession of Christianity, that is, of what is most perfect in moral discipline and legal principle, in the presence of the entire past company, among the most enlightened nations, of men versed in the science of civil and religious legislation, that "what marriage in itself is was previously unknown"—marriage, this element of every society, this *contract* which is truly *social,* the founding act of the family, whose laws are the basis for all political legislation? How could one assert that "it is only *in recent times* that men have acquired precise ideas on marriage"? And from when do these *recent times* date? Is it from the time of Luther, who allowed the dissolution of marriage, or from that of modern philosophy, which, not content to allow the easiest dissolution of the conjugal tie, has justified concubinage and extended its indulgence to adultery? And does it not already prejudge the issue in favor of the utility of divorce to assert, in the preamble of the law authorizing it, that *what marriage is was unknown until recent times?*

"Marriage as it existed before the establishment of Christianity, which preceded all positive law, and which derives

discussion, a revised version of this code was adopted in 1804, often called the *Code Napoléon,* which still serves as the basis for French law, as well as for that of several Latin American countries and the state of Louisiana.

from the very constitution of our being, is neither a civil nor a religious act, but a natural one, which attracted the attention of the legislator, and which religion has consecrated." *Marriage existed before Christianity, and preceded all positive law;* but did it precede the natural relationships between sociable beings, of which the Christian religion offers the most perfect development, and of which all religious and political laws are merely the expression and manifestation?

The sentence just cited is highly misleading, and the various meanings it appears to present vanish under scrutiny.

Marriage is civil in terms of interests, religious in terms of souls; it is *animal* or physical in terms of bodies; and as the family has never, at any time whatever, been able to survive without property, and as man has always entered into marriage with all of his moral and physical capacities, it is accurate to say that marriage, in itself and at bottom, has always been a civil, religious, and physical act at once. It was not a civil act in the earliest times, in the sense that the interests of the family were defended by public force and ruled by public laws, which constitute what we call the *civil state;* but they were defended by domestic power, element of public power, and were ruled by morals or domestic laws, seeds of public laws, just as domestic society, or the family, is itself the element and seed of public society. Marriage was not religious in the sense that there were priests to bless it, but in the sense that it was divine, and that the Creator had said of woman, "She will leave her father and mother and cleave unto her husband," and of the spouses, "They will be two in one flesh." It is because marriage, in the earliest times and prior to the establishment of public, political, and religious societies, was a divine and human act (I understand by a human act a moral and physical one), as, ever since the establishment of public societies, it has been a civil and religious act; that is why, I say, it derives from the constitution of our being, of our nature, and is a *natural* act: for the true nature of man and the real constitution of his being consist in natural relationships with his being's author, and in natural relationships, both moral and physical, with his fellows. It is only because marriage was both divine and human in the sense I mean that it *attracted the attention* of the civil legislator, and was consecrated by religion; for if the orator whose reasoning I am discussing, who opposes the *natural* to the civil and religious, as if what is civil and religious were not natural, understands by nature man's animality, he falls into the same error as the Council of State's reporter for the section of the Civil Code on marriage, when he says that "philosophers consider in marriage only the proximity of the sexes." These are certainly, to mention it in passing, some strange philosophers; and it seems that only anatomists are thus allowed to consider the union of man and woman.

Natural marriage, which is *neither civil nor religious,* gives birth to Jean-Jacques Rousseau's *natural* man, who is himself neither *civil* nor *religious;* and to say that marriage is *neither a civil nor a religious act, but a natural one* is to assert that the civil and religious states are not in man's nature, and to fall back into the doctrine of the writer just mentioned when he says that "society is not in man's nature"; and elsewhere: "everything that is not in nature has its disadvantages, and civil society more than all the rest."

Let us say, then, that marriage is at once a social, domestic, civil, and religious act; the founding act of domestic society, whose interests should be guaranteed by civil authority, coming to the aid of domestic harmony, and in which religious authority causes Divinity to intervene in an external and sensible manner, in order to consecrate the union of hearts and purify the union of bodies.

The principle of the Civil Code's author is erroneous, but consistent, and he was obliged to deny the civil and religious bond of marriage, which he wished to dissolve by civil authority, to the prejudice of religious authority.

I believe that, in the principles I have just set forth, one can

find a satisfactory solution to the celebrated question debated
in the school, namely: Whether the essence of marriage consists in the mutual faith of the spouses, or in the sacrament
conferred by the Church. If one considers marriage in the
purely domestic state of society, as it necessarily existed in the
earliest times, or as it would still exist, and just as necessarily,
between two human beings of different sexes cast away on a
desert island, then marriage consists in the mutual faith of the
spouses; if one considers it among Christians living in the
public state of religious society, then it consists in the union of
hearts, ratified and consecrated by the sacrament; and the
opposite decision, even if handed down with good intentions,
reflects the spirit of the century, and may have dangerous
consequences.

Be that as it may, no question is simpler in its principles or
more fertile in its consequences than that of divorce, since by
itself it raises all the fundamental questions for society concerning *power* and *duty;* and I do not hesitate to affirm, and I
even hope to show, that on the dissolubility or indissolubility
of the conjugal tie depends, in France and everywhere, the fate
of the family, religion, and the State.

In 1789, the family would have been saved from destruction
if the political constitution had been defended against democracy; today, to save the State, the domestic constitution must
be defended against divorce; a cruel capacity, which takes all
authority from the father, all dignity from the mother, all security from the child, and transforms domestic society into a
struggle between strength and weakness, between *power* and
duty; which constitutes the family as a temporary lease, where
the inconstancy of the human heart stipulates its passions and
interests, and which ends where other interests and new passions begin.

Divorce was decreed in 1792, and it came as no surprise,
because it was an inevitable *consequence,* long foreseen, of the
system of destruction followed at that time with such ardor;

but today, when one seeks to rebuild, divorce enters the foundations of the social edifice as a *principle;* and this must cause severe apprehension among those destined to inhabit it.

I will go further. Divorce was in harmony with democracy, which reigned too long in France under various names and forms. Domestic power on the one hand, and public power on the other, were delivered up to the passions of the subjects; there was disorder in the family and disorder in the State: between the two, there was a parity and an analogy of disorder. And there is, so to speak, some sort of order where everything is disordered in the same manner and sense. But divorce is directly contradictory to the spirit and principles of hereditary or indissoluble monarchy. There is then order in the State and disorder in the family; indissolubility in the one, dissolubility in the other, a lack of harmony in consequence; and in this situation, either the family must end by disordering the State, or the State by ordering the family. There is more. In a democracy, the people has the privilege of making laws and abolishing them according to its whims. But because of the short duration of its magistracies, it is rare for there to be individuals powerful enough to bend the laws to their passions; whereas in monarchy, where eminent positions, granted for life or hereditarily, give rise to great powers and fortunes, it can happen that the laws are, not made, but interpreted according to the wishes of the most influential persons; and what judgments are solicited by more lively passions than judgments in divorce, and what laws better lend themselves to arbitrary interpretation than those which limit or extend its faculty? Now, where the great have passed, the crowd passes in turn. What was difficult becomes easy, what was rare becomes common, what was forbidden becomes allowed; the exception acquires the force of law, soon the law is reduced to an exception; and the time comes when there is no longer any remedy for disorder but disorder carried to an extreme, or revolutions.

The jurist sees a contract in marriage; the publicist sees a

society in the family, and the first of societies. It is from the
latter standpoint alone that I consider the question of divorce.
I leave it to others to discuss the proposed Civil Code's arrangements concerning the possession and transmission of
property; here I shall treat only the relationships between
persons.

In this discussion, I shall use only the eloquence of reason,
because I speak to legislators, and in the presence of a nation
which, through force of experience, has arrived at that state in
which it is easier to convince than to sweep along. Moreover, if
the imagination paints the deplorable effects of divorce in
more vivid colors, it presents just as lively a picture of the too
often unhappy results of indissoluble unions; and in this uncertain contest, truth triumphs only by the accident of talent. Let
us give its success a more certain chance, by fighting for it with
its own weapons, which error cannot use without betraying its
weakness.

I shall not even seek motives against divorce in the private affections of man, affections which are fleeting and
changeable, and often directed toward culpable objects, more
vivid sometimes than legitimate ones. The reason for man's
duties, like the reward for his virtues, must be sought outside
of man himself. The man, woman, and children are indissolubly *united* not because their hearts must take pleasure in this
union—for then how would we answer those for whom this
union is a torment?—but because a natural law makes it a duty
for them, and because universal reason, from which this law
emanates, has founded society on a base less fragile than the
affections of man.

I invite the reader to reread the part of the introduction to
the proposed Civil Code which deals with marriage and the
faculty of divorce. He will note, in its contradictory presenta-
tion of reasons for and against divorce, that the advantage lies
wholly with the cause of indissolubility, and indeed that there
reigns in this regard a striking contradiction between the gen-

eral spirit of the introduction and the text of the Code. This observation has escaped no one. Some have attributed it to the inherent superiority of the cause, others to the personal opinions of the authors, and all were right. In this instance the authors' minds were in agreement with their hearts; but such is the dominion of former times over the present that, in this unpleasant task, they were allowed to follow neither their sentiments nor their opinions. The public has recognized in particular the superior talent which M. Portalis, the *vir bonus dicendi peritus* of Cicero,[2] deployed on the days of battle in this same cause, as in others of no less importance. One is grateful to know him at the same time one is called to combat him, because one feels more keenly the advantage of agreeing with the intentions of the man, in the very places that one does share the opinions of the author.

I shall be forced to recall the religious beliefs of the part of the nation which rejects divorce, solely because the proposed Civil Code makes reference to the religious beliefs of the part of the nation which accepts its faculty; for, moreover, I think that on this question the government should concern itself, not with religious beliefs, but with reasonable actions; and it will doubtless be noticed that if I cite the Christian religion in support of my arguments, it is to show its conformity with the most enlightened reason, and not at all to seek motives in it capable of subjugating reason.

[2] "A good man skilled in speaking." Cato the Censor, from the fragment. Seneca the Elder,

CHAPTER 2

Of Domestic Society

MAN and woman both *are;* but they *are* not both the same or in an equal manner, and they differ in sex.

This equality in being, this inequality in manner of being, is called *similarity,* and constitutes beings which are *similar* but not *equal,* and which can never become equal.

The union of the sexes is the reason for their difference; the production of a being is the purpose of their union.

The being produced is of the same sex as one or the other of those that gave it being; but they are formed and it is to be formed; it is young and they are old. Another inequality, another similarity.

Man, woman, *little one,* considered each in itself, and without any relation between them, each form an *individual,* that is to say, a whole which cannot be divided without destroying it. Their ways of being, of sex, and of age are *absolute,* which is to say that these ways exist independently of one another; for in an organized being, *young* is not relative to *old;* and the organized being is, in an absolute sense, young as long as it is growing, and old when it is diminishing.

Father, mother, child, which express both the union of the sexes and the production of the being, can only be considered dependently on one another, and relatively to one another. A woman could exist without the existence of a man; but there is no mother if there is no father, nor a child without both of them. Each one of these ways of being presumes and recalls the other two; that is to say, they are *relative*. Considered thus,

42

they are called *relationships*, in Latin, *ratio;* father, mother, child are *persons*, and their union forms the family. The union of the sexes, which is the foundation of all these relationships, is called *marriage*.

Thus the similarity of human beings has produced relationships between them; as the similarity of material beings, considered in the spatial sense, produces arithmetic or geometric relationships; as the similarity of material beings, considered in their substance, produces *affinities* or chemical relationships. These points of contact between the various sciences are precious to collect.

The production of man is the purpose of the relationship between the sexes; his conservation is the purpose of the relationship between the ages, which is to say that man and woman produce the child, and the father and mother conserve it. The production and conservation of man are thus the purpose of the family, and the reason for all the relationships of sex and age which constitute it.

The beast is born with an impulsion, according to some, with a knowledge, according to others; an impulsion or a knowledge which is called *instinct*, which guides each species invariably and all species infallibly in their reproduction and conservation, for which purposes each has received everything it needs. The beast is no more free not to reproduce itself than not to conserve itself. Time, manner, everything is determined for it; and whatever our lessons add to its instinct is always for our needs rather than its own, and demonstrates its industriousness much less than ours.

Man, on the contrary, is born ignorant and helpless; and if the faculty of choosing and willing which distinguishes him were not enlightened by instruction, he would have no choice; he would have an impulsion but no will, movements but no action. He would accede to certain involuntary needs, but he would be unable either to foresee danger or to protect himself from it. Unable to conserve and perhaps to reproduce himself,* he would be lower than the beast, or rather he would be nothing, because he would not be what he must be, and because, unlike the beast, he has not received an instinct to take the place of his will.

Man is therefore not, as M. de Saint-Lambert says, "an organized and sensible mass, which receives spirit from everything in its environment and from its needs"; but man is *an intelligence served by organs, which receive from* their form and from instruction a disposition to second the intelligence in the exercise of his will and the control of his action.†

The *means* of this instruction is speech; for man in society never acts without a *means, medium,* or *mediator*—words which are absolutely synonymous.

Speech, which expresses the thought of the father in order to form the thought of the son, to teach him to will, and consequently to act, is known to the father, unknown to the son; for indeed it was only possible to designate the little one of the human race by saying "he who does not speak," *infans.*[2]

Thus in the conservation or instruction of man, as in his reproduction, the father is active or strong, the child passive or weak; while the mother, *median term between the two extremes of this continuous proportion, is passive* to conceive, active to produce, receives to transmit, learns to teach, and obeys to command.

*The men of the two sexes, outside all society, without language, and hence without reason, would flee each other, fight each other, and not unite. What shows this is that the passion of love is weaker in man the closer he is to the barbarous state, and stronger in the beast the closer it is to life in the wild. All the men found in the woods have shown indifference to women, and vice versa.

†*Tantum abest ut corpus quoquo modo sui juris sit,* says the celebrated Stahl, *ut potius alterius sit juris, animae inquam, et intelligendi ac volendi actui ministret.*[1]

[1] "So far is the body from ruling itself in any way that rather it is itself ruled by something else, I mean by the soul, and serves the act of understanding and willing."

[2] "One who does not speak."

This gradation in their relationships—in which alone lies the solution to the divorce question—is marked in a sensible manner even in the beings' purely physical relations. Man, gifted with knowledge, is a father only by will; woman, even with knowledge, can become a mother in spite of her will; the child has neither the will to be born nor the knowledge that it is being born.

This necessary cooperation of the mother in the father's action for the child, this dual relationship which unites her to both of them, and from which it ensues that, in her body as in her spirit, the woman partakes of the strength of the one and the weakness of the other, is called *means* or *ministry*.

Thus one can say that "the father has, or is, the *power* to accomplish, through the means or *ministry* of the mother, the reproductive and conservative action of which the child is the term or *subject*."

If I may be allowed to discard, as in an analysis, the expression of the physical relationships, *father, mother, child*, which apply to the beast as well as to man, then we shall have the expression *power, minister, subject*, related like *father, mother, child*—an expression of the moral relationships which only apply to the intelligent being, but which apply to all intelligent beings, embrace the generality, the immensity of their relationships, and open the very gates of the infinite to contemplation.

Father, mother, child were the physical persons; their relationships were physical, and formed the animal family; *power, minister, subject* are the moral or social persons, or simply the *persons;** their relationships are moral or social, and form the

Person comes from *per se sonat*,[3] which in itself expresses a social relation. *Paul* is a word which designates an individual but enounces no particular quality. *Power, minister, subject* are *persons;* that is to say, they express relationships by themselves, *per se sonant*, but designate no particular individual.
[3] "It sounds by itself."

moral family, or the society which is called domestic, *a domo,*[4] because community of dwelling is one of its necessary conditions.

I insist intentionally on these moral expressions which designate the domestic persons for several reasons:

1. Because, since the expressions father, mother, and child present only relationships of sex and age, the modern sophists have abused them, in order to consider us as merely males, females, and young, and because it is necessary in a sense to spiritualize man and his relationships, in proportion to the efforts made to materialize them.

2. Because the expressions *power, minister,* and *subject* carry the enunciation of their functions and of the duties of each member of society.

3. Because these general expressions, current in public society, exhibit its similarity to domestic society, and simplify the development of their common principles.

The Christian religion itself, which I shall never cite in the course of this work except to show its conformity with reason, calls man the *reason,* the *head,* the *power* of woman: *Vir caput est mulieris,*[5] says Saint Paul. It calls woman the helper or *minister*[6] of man: "Let us make man," says Genesis, "a helper similar to him." It calls the child a *subject,* since it tells it, in a thousand places, to obey its parents.

The family thus acquired a character of morality, and this is what the author of the introduction to the proposed Civil Code says in different terms: "When a nation is formed, there is more concern with the dignity of marriage than with its purpose."

Man's malice always increases; that is to say, man tends, by a penchant he is born with, to exaggerate his power, woman to

---

[4] "From 'the house.'"
[5] "Man is the head of woman." Paul, 1 Corinthians 11.3.
[6] "Helper."

usurp it, the child to escape it. This inclination, whatever its cause, is an indisputable fact.

Religion thus merely informs us of a fact when it teaches us that we are all born with an original or native penchant for domination, called *pride;* a penchant which betrays our natural magnitude, and for which society is the restraint, because society includes the institutions which maintain legitimate power, conservative of beings, against men's passions, and is nothing but the protection of weakness against the abuse of strength; and modern philosophy denies both truth and reason when it says, by the voice of Jean-Jacques Rousseau, that "man is born good, and society depraves him."

The physical strength of the father could not contain this penchant for independence in the other family members; for several children are stronger than a father, and a man's very life is at every moment at his wife's disposition.

What bond, then, will hold the domestic persons in the place assigned them by their duties? The *natural affections,* say the sophists, who do not fail to cite as evidence the affections of the beasts; *sympathy,* say novelists; *sentiment,* say *sensible* souls. But if these affections are natural to us, like the need to digest and to sleep, why are there unjust fathers, ungrateful children, unfaithful wives, unkind brothers? Why have laws, when there are necessities? Is this pretended natural affection for others not too often ready to give way to affection for oneself? And far from being natural, does it never require efforts against themselves for spouses to stay united, and for children to remain obedient? These natural affections are therefore merely reasonable ones, which habit, gratitude, and above all self-love make dear, easy, and sometimes blind; and if they are reasonable affections, then they are reasoned or learned. For man is born capable of reason; but he learns to reason, and does not reason unless he has learned to do so. Thus one can say that the reason for all our reasonable affections, or for all our duties, is found only in reason.

The child receives reason from its parents by the communication of speech, as it received being from them by the communication of life. Its parents in turn received both of these from those who preceded them. The noticeable progression of population, wherever it is not thwarted by accidental or local causes, demonstrates, like every geometric progression, a generative first term. Every people, and humankind itself, was born from a family, since it could still begin anew from a family if that family alone remained in the universe. Hence in the infancy of the world, the peoples were known only by the names of families: the children of Eber, of Moab, of Edom, *Dardaniae, Pelasgi,* etc.

Was this first family born of the earth or the sea, the sun or the moon? It has been said in this century, in which the fables of Prometheus and Deucalion have been revived. But why do the elements today produce nothing comparable? If we could be shown an insect born without father or mother, from matter in fermentation, then we could believe in the formation of man by matter. Let us therefore say, with reason and history, that an intelligent being produced the intelligent being. And that, if we do not understand the mystery of this divine generation, we understand no better the mystery of human generation, because everything in the universe, including man himself, is a mystery for man. Thus we *imagine* effects, such as fluidity, the force of the wind, gravity, adhesion, etc., without *conceiving* them; and we *conceive* their cause without *imagining* it. For the proposition *there is no effect without a cause* is as evident to reason as the proposition *there is no body without space* is certain to the imagination.

This being, author of man, and therefore superior to him, as the cause is to the effect, is called *God,* and it is even an absurdity to say that man invented God; for to invent a being would be to create it, and man can no more create beings than he can destroy them. He develops their relationships, he alters their forms: these are the limits of his invention and action;

and one can defy all the philosophers together to invent something of which men had no previous idea, as to draw a figure which does not lie inside already known dimensions.

In God is thus the reason for creation; in God is the reason for conservation, which is a continued creation.

If God made man, then there is in God, as in man, *intelligence* which willed, *action* which executed. There is thus similarity, and *man is made in his image and likeness.* There are thus relationships, a society; and I see, throughout the universe, religion as soon as the family, and the society of man and God as soon as the society of man and man; this primitive religion is called *natural* or *domestic*.

But if man today receives speech as he receives being; if he speaks only insofar as he hears speech, and speaks only the language he hears spoken; if it is even physically impossible for man to invent speech by himself, as it is impossible for him to invent being by himself (which can be shown by considering the operations of thought and those of the vocal organ), then it is necessary that man in the beginning received speech and being together. Now this truth, which would be an even physical demonstration of the existence of a first being, though combatted, or rather misunderstood, by the sophists, is little by little establishing itself in society; and already Jean-Jacques Rousseau had said: "Overwhelmed by the difficulties which present themselves" (in the discussion of Condillac's novel on the *invention of language*),[7] "and convinced of the nearly proven impossibility that languages could have arisen and established themselves by purely human means, I leave the discussion of this difficult problem to anyone who cares to undertake the task . . . and I believe that speech was very necessary to invent speech."

It is, in effect, these last words which present the reason for

[7] A reference to the abbé Etienne Bonnot de Condillac's *Essai sur l'origine des connaissances humaines* (Amsterdam: P. Mortier, 1746; various subsequent editions).

the impossibility of the invention of language by men: for to invent is to think, and to think is to speak inside oneself. Signs are required for thought, because they are required for speech; and one can say, to summarize, that *man thinks his speech before speaking his thought,* and expresses his thought for himself before expressing it for others.

Human reason is in divine speech, as the child's reason is in the father's speech. That is why *speech* and *reason* are expressed in Greek by the same word, *logos;* and man could not have reasoned by himself, since he could not have even spoken by himself; and if I do not understand the incomprehensible mystery of human speech, why should I seek to penetrate the mystery of divine speech?

The society between God and primitive man has all the general characteristics of the society we have observed between men, and I see in it the moral persons: the *power,* who is God; the *subjects,* who are the domestic persons; the *minister,* who is the father of the family; a median too between the *two extremes of this continuous proportion:* "God is to the father as the father is to the child." The father is at once passive and active, partaking of the dependence of the child and the power of God himself; receiving orders to transmit them, and obeying one to command the other.

And nowhere do I find a historical truth better established than the religion of the first families and the priesthood of the first patriarchs.

In this domestic cult of Divinity, the mother had a distinguished place, or perhaps some function relative to her rank in the family. Hence the priestesses of pagan religion, and hence the usual tendency of ancient peoples, whose traces can still be seen in modern times, to attribute something superhuman to women, and in particular knowledge of the future. *Inesse quin etiam feminis sanctum aliquid et providum putant,* says Tacitus, speaking of the Germans.[8]

[8] "Moreover, they believe that there is something sacred and prophetic in women." Tacitus, *Germany* 8.2.

Thus the existence of man demonstrates the creation of beings, and the existence of the family demonstrates the conservation of man; hence it demonstrates the knowledge of the natural relationships of men in the family, which are the only means of conservation; of instruction, which is the only means of knowledge; of speech, which is the only means of instruction; of God, finally, who alone knows by himself the relationships of the beings he has created, and who alone can reveal them to men.

This speech which teaches the natural relationships is called *law.* The law is thus the enunciation of the natural relationships between the persons—a truth universally recognized from Cicero, who said, *Lex est ratio profecta a natura rerum,*[9] to Jean-Jacques Rousseau, who said, "Natural relationships and laws must always agree on the same points."

It is from the sentiment of this truth that the ancient legislators called laws the thought of God, *mentem Dei,* says Cicero,[10] and that Jean-Jacques Rousseau called laws the speech of God: "What God wills man to do," he says, "he does not tell him through another man, he tells it to him himself, and writes it at the bottom of his heart." And the true philosopher, who senses that this fanatical opinion* is the theory of all extravagances and the arsenal of all crimes, sets reality in place of metaphor, completes the thought of Cicero, rectifies that of Jean-Jacques Rousseau; believes, with the

---

*Fanaticism consists in believing that God perpetually acts without means, like a prince who, relying on God for the care of his defense by a supernatural operation, neglects to levy troops. Superstition consists in believing that God always acts through means unrelated to their end, *verbis, herbis, lapidibus,*[11] says Cagliostro. Enthusiasm or zeal is good or bad, depending on its end and its means.

[9] "The law is a relationship which derives from the nature of things." This passage has not been found in Cicero. Somewhat similar passages are found in Cicero, *On the Laws* 1.6 and 1.15.

[10] "The thought of God." Cicero, *Tusculan Disputations* 1.66.

[11] "By means of words, herbs, and stones."

former, in a divine thought; with the latter, in a divine speech, but a speech given to a man for men, a real speech, which man can hear if he is willing to listen to it. This is what made Charles Bonnet say that "the (revealed) law is an even *physical* expression of the will of God."

Thus, *love God, honor your father and mother* must have been the first words *spoken* to the family, as later they were the first words *written* for a people; and then God, power, functions, duties, everything was revealed to man, and the father of the family had only to transmit this knowledge and command its execution.

"It was above all through the patriarchs' relationships to society," says the estimable author of the *Historical Essay on Paternal Power*,*[12] "that the father's power grew in the earliest times. Little by little his wishes were confused with those of which religious worship made him the voice. Thus was formed that general opinion of heroic times which attributed to them a supernatural influence on the elements and destiny. This influence placed all the attributes of divine justice in his hands." From this arose, according to the same author, the paternal curse, or domestic excommunication, which imparted a terror so deep it has lasted across the centuries to our own times.

Hence it is in divine power alone that the Christian religion finds the reason for domestic laws. "Husbands," it says, "love your wives as the Lord loved his Church, and gave himself for her; wives, be submissive to your husbands as to God; children, obey your parents in the Lord."

Thus man owes nothing to man except for God and in the sight of God: therein lies the true equality and true *liberty of the children of God,* to which Christianity raises us; and all human duty ends at the point where divine power is no longer recognized.

*M. André Nougarède.
[12] André-Jean-Simon, baron Nougarède de Fayet, *Essai sur l'histoire de la puissance paternelle et sur le divorce* (Paris: Le Normant, Year IX [1801]).

Thus domestic physical laws are the enunciation of the relationships of the father, mother, and child; and domestic moral laws, which are also called morals, are the enunciation of the relationships of the moral persons: of the power, minister, and subject.

Thus every family in which the father cannot cease to be a power, the mother to be subordinate, the son to be dependent, will have good laws or good morals; and the family will have bad laws or bad morals when the moral persons can cease to be in their respective relationships.

Thus domestic morals are different from individual morals, or the conduct of the individual; for man can be disordered in a well-ordered society, or ordered himself in a society which is not. In one case, man is better than society; in the other, society is better than man.

Thus *love God, honor your father and mother* is the fundamental law of the family, of which the subsequent domestic laws must be the result: a natural or true result where God is *served* and the father obeyed; a false and unnatural result where God is outraged by a false worship and domestic power undermined by senseless laws.

Thus religion is the bond of domestic persons, the bond between God and men, the bond of intelligent beings: *a religare,* to bind doubly.*

*See the *First Laws,* by the same author, where these truths are developed in detail.

CHAPTER 3

Of Public Society

MEN multiply, and families live nearer one another. Common needs bring them together, but equally strong passions more often disunite them. Women, children, herds, territories, hunting and fishing grounds—everything becomes a subject of conflict between families. In every society, and indeed in every age of society, there are private wars as soon as there are families living close together; and neighbors who sue each other today would have taken up arms a few centuries ago.

The domestic state is necessary to reproduce and conserve man: he makes himself a public state, or political government, to multiply and conserve families. In effect, in all times and among all peoples, I perceive a man who speaks and commands, and men who listen and obey—that is to say, men in an active state and men in a passive one; I perceive other men (magistrates or warriors), *median between the two extremes,* located at an equal distance between the power and the subjects, who receive the orders they transmit, and obey to command.

Not only do I perceive this order in the universe, but reason tells me that this order is natural, that it cannot be otherwise for the conservation of families; that there must be a general will to give a common action to all wills, and a general action to prevent the collision of particular actions; and if this order is shown to be necessary, I shall care little whether it is voluntary or forced in its principle,* and I see no contract where I see a necessity.

I perceive, then, a human power, ministers, and subjects, who are not fathers, mothers, or children, considered in terms of physical relationship; but who, having the multiplication and conservation of families as the end of their relations, present an end *similar* to that of the family, whose object is the reproduction and conservation of man, and who thus have a general or public end, as the family has a particular and domestic one.

From this similarity in means and ends arises a similarity in names. Power, in every religious and political society, is called *paternity*, and subjects are called *children;* and this is what made the author of the introduction to the Civil Code say that "magistrates are fathers wherever fathers are magistrates."

In domestic society or the family, the power is a man, it is *one;* and in the public or general society called the State, the power must be a man, and he is always *one*, appearances to the contrary notwithstanding; for *one* man alone proposes the law which all accept; indeed, often *one* alone decides when many deliberate. Every legislative assembly is divided by *one* seat; and the only difference in this regard between the most unlimited democracy and hereditary monarchy is that unity is fixed in the latter, and perpetually mobile in the former.

In the family, which is a society of individuals, the power, minister, and subject are in the individual; in the State, which is a society of families, the power, minister, and subject are often in the family. The families of the public ministry are

---

*Plato, in his *Republic*, also considers three orders of citizens, the judges, warriors, and artisans; but the judges and warriors form a single person in society, since they are merely the internal and external means of society's conservation. To this distinction of social persons corresponds that of the cardinal virtues. Prudence belongs to the head, strength to the minister, temperance or modesty to the subject, justice to all; for it conserves all relationships.

called *notables* or nobles. Sometimes the power alone is in the family, as in Turkey; sometimes the ministry alone, as in Poland; in some cases, the power and the ministry are in the same families, which are called *patrician,* as in aristocracies and oligarchies; in other cases, everything is in individuals, as in democracies.

In the family, the persons, laws, functions, duties, and virtues are domestic or private; in the State, everything is public—persons, laws, functions, duties, and virtues.

Public society has not destroyed or even altered the relationships of domestic society, since the child is a minor or subject in the family, even when he has reached his majority in the State; and since the father is a subject in the State, even though he holds the power in the family. Once the public State is formed, domestic power is clearly distinguished from physical paternity: (1) since this power exists even where paternity is only presumed, following this axiom of the law: *Pater est is quem justae nuptiae demonstrant;*[1] (2) since even when the father has ceased to be, the power continues in his last wishes, and even in perpetuity in the case of entails; (3) since the power exists even where paternity does not, as when the firstborn succeeds to the power of a deceased father over the latter's children; (4) the power is transmissible, and paternity is not, as when a father appoints a guardian for his young sons. Public power, which is also called political when it administers the State, and civil when it rules families, regards the mother solely as a domestic person and her husband's *minister,* since she must be authorized by him for all civil acts in which she intervenes.

The passions which trouble the family are far more violent in the State, because, at the same time that they are inflamed by ambition for public power, they are not dampened by the influence of the domestic affections.

---

[1] "The man indicated by a regular marriage is the father."

The human power cannot keep the ministers and subjects in their places by himself, because he is one against all, and the weapons he gives them for his defense can be turned against him.

Here the universal bond of every society, religion, comes once more to strengthen the ties of political society, and the very word religion, from *religare,* sufficiently proclaims that it is the natural and necessary bond of human societies, families, and States. Religion, from being domestic, becomes public or revealed; as society, from being domestic, has become public State or government; and if families without a domestic religion are nowhere to be found in the earliest times, there has yet to be a public State of society without a public or revealed religion; for the Moslem religion is a religion revealed or taught by Mohammed, as the Christian religion was revealed by Jesus Christ.*

The persons of domestic or natural religion were internal or domestic: the minister, the subjects, the power itself. This is attested by Scripture, sole monument of the earliest ages of the world, where we see the heads of families as sacrificers, priests, in a word *ministers* of a God who protected their families, and who himself wished to be called the *God of Abraham,* the *God of Isaac,* the *God of Jacob.*

In public or revealed religion, the persons become public. The subjects are the nation, the ministers are the priesthood, *median between two extremes,* in communication with God and with man, receiving to transmit, and obeying one to prescribe to the others. Very Divinity makes itself external, in a sense, and *present:* in a *sensible* manner, in the Judaic tabernacle from which it rendered its oracles; in a *real* manner, on the

---

*Among Christians this expression, *revealed religion,* refers solely to a divine revelation, or the manifestation of truth; but in the proper acceptation in which I use it here, *to reveal* means to teach, to discover, *revelare,* and one senses well enough that it is in this sense alone that I compare Mohammed and Jesus Christ, or error and truth.

altars of the Christian religion; and even the pagans represent
it in a *material* or *figurative* manner in the idols of their gods.
The major act of religious worship, man's gift or the sacrifice,
which is internal in domestic religion, is also public in public
society, and even blood-soaked in pagan religion.

The laws become public, like the persons whose relationships they enunciate. The law to *honor the father and
mother*, fundamental to domestic society, becomes fundamental to public society; and it is the sentiment of M. Bossuet that
the obligation to obey political power and its agents lies in this
precept.

Only religion can therefore prevent the displacement of the
public persons, as it prevents the displacement of the domestic
ones. This truth was known to the sages of antiquity when they
wished to found societies, and to our modern sages when they
wished to destroy them, since the former began by regulating
the worship of Divinity, and the latter by abolishing it.

And note that here the result is found alongside the principle, and that after the law which commands man to *honor*
power and its ministers, the legislator adds: *so that you may
live long on earth,* because the natural constitution of domestic and public power ensures the longevity of families and the
perpetuity of empires. Montesquieu attributes the tranquillity
of modern States to the Christian religion; and history, more
instructive in its lessons than philosophy in its science, shows
us non-Christian societies declining as they move away from
their origins, and tending toward their decadence even when
they push back their frontiers; and Christian society in general
becoming, from age to age, more enlightened and strong, and
drawing new enlightenment and strength even from revolutions.

Thus the reason for public power is in divine power, and can
be found nowhere else. Man naturally has no dominion over
man, man owes nothing to man; all power constituted on

natural or divine laws comes from God, *omnis potestas ex Deo*,[2] and this passage has never been understood otherwise.

Thus, political power is the means or minister of divine power for the conservation of the human species, which is inseparably bound up with the existence of society; *minister Dei in bonum*, says Saint Paul:[3] *median also between two extremes*, God and man; and political power thus finds in the law of God the basis for the secondary laws which it publishes to rule men, and obeys one to command the others. For as soon as one does not deny the existence of Divinity, one must either renounce the act of reasoning or accept this series of consequences.

Thus, once legitimate power comes from God, authority is justified and obedience ennobled, and man must equally fear to command and be honored to obey.

One sees why, among the earliest peoples, the priesthood and the kingship were united; why, among the Romans, a member of the priestly college who was charged with offering the national sacrifice bore the title *king;* and finally why, in modern nations, Christian princes, like the Hebrew kings, receive a special consecration, and have even been called *the external bishops.*

Language, an expression of social man, began with man and has perfected itself along with society. The difference between the sexes is expressed in substantives; the distinction between persons, in verbs; the type of domestic or public society, in singular or plural numbers, *I, thou,* or *we;* of which the former are reserved for the speech of the family, the latter for public power; and the very constitution of society, formed by a power, a subject, and a minister, each the bond of the other, is found revealed in the construction of the sentence, formed by a governor, a governed, and a binding-word, either verb or cop-

[2] "All power is from God." Paul, Romans 13.1.
[3] "God's servant for what is good." Paul, Romans 13.4.

ula, which unites them to each other; relationships which are all the more remarkable in that the order of these three parts of all human discourse, called syntax, is natural or *analogous* in societies which are naturally constituted, and *inverted* or *transpositive* in societies which are not. I shall stop here: this theory of discourse, considered as an expression of social man, would carry me too far from the subject at hand; I reserve for other occasions its developments, which concern the most important social and even literary truths.

The principles just discussed lead to two practical results whose utility will not escape the reader.

1. The first is that, in his social state, the intelligent being only acts mediately and through means, ministers, medians, mediators, intermediaries; for all these expressions are synonymous. This proposition,* seriously considered and developed in all its aspects, could teach certain philosophers that modern philosophy's case against religion, which they believe to be decided beyond appeal, and irretrievably lost for the Christians, has hardly begun, and that the parties have, so to speak, as yet only argued the question of competence, because some wished to bring the case before the tribunal of reason, while others appealed to the tribunal of faith. There still remain very weighty considerations to be set forth in favor of religion; "for," Charles Bonnet says very well, "all moral truths are enfolded within one another, and from this, reflection is sooner or later able to extract them."

But the time has perhaps not yet come to set forth these great truths in all of their majesty: one can at most indicate them to attentive minds. There are two periods in the life of a nation when one must fear to tax its weakness with overly serious and prolonged instruction: the first, when one soothes its childhood with fairy tales; the second, when one lulls its decrepitude with licentious writings and absurd systems,

---

*It is developed in the *First Laws*.

which retard the progress of man's reason, by all that they do to hasten the development of his passions.

2. The other conclusion which follows from the principles we have presented is that, since the family is the element of the State, and the State is the development of the family, and since these two societies are *similar* in their constitutions, any change that occurs will be reciprocal between them, and any displacement of persons in one will produce a displacement of persons in the other.

Thus polygamy, which is domestic despotism, strengthens and maintains political despotism wherever it is practiced, as in Turkey, China, Persia, etc. When political power in Poland, upon the extinction of the Jagiellon dynasty, was seized by a powerful aristocracy and fell from its primitive constitution, receiving that unruly form which has prolonged its weakness and caused its ruin, marriage ceased to be as respected as in other Catholic States; and it is this alone which has led a number of persons to believe, and to assert to a number of others, that divorce is allowed in Poland.

Having set forth the constitutional principles of domestic society and of public society, we have now acquired enough information to treat the question of marriage, which, among civilized peoples, is both a domestic and a public act.

CHAPTER 4

Of Marriage

MARRIAGE is the commitment made by two people of different sexes to unite in order to form a society called the family.

Modern philosophy give marriage a different end. In the chimerical state of perfection which Condorcet, in his posthumous work on the *Progress of the Human Mind,*[1] supposes that men will someday attain—thus attributing to the individual the perfection which should be in society—"men," he says, "will then understand that if they have any obligation to beings which do not yet exist, it cannot be to give them existence": a notion which rings false, expressed in a ridiculous sentence, and wholly on a par with the statement of the soldier who, ordered to carry out a rigorous execution, replied to an unfortunate begging for his life, "My friend, ask me for anything you like, except life."

The union of all with all indiscriminately is the *promiscuity* of the beasts; the successive union of one with many is polygamy, repudiation, divorce; the indissoluble union of one with one was Christian marriage formerly, and Catholic marriage today: all these forms of marriage can thus be reduced to the unity of union and the multiplicity of unions.

Thus, as *promiscuity* is the union of the most imperfect of living beings, the beasts, it appears that indissoluble union, which is the other extreme, must be the union of the most perfect of living beings, men; and that the states intermediate

[1] Marie-Jean-Antoine-Nicolas de Caritat, marquis de Condorcet, *Esquisse d'un tableau historique des progrès de l'esprit humain* (Paris: Agasse, Year III [1794–1795]).

between these two states will be more or less perfect insofar as they approach one or the other: a universally recognized truth, since the adversaries of indissolubility only criticize it for its perfection.

If human marriage is a union with a commitment to form a society, it differs essentially from concubinage, which is a union without a commitment to form a society, and still more from vague libertinism, which is a union with an intention not to form a society.

The end of marriage is therefore not the happiness of the spouses, if by happiness one understands an idyllic pleasure of the heart and senses, which the man who loves independence finds far more readily in unions without a commitment.

Religion and the State consider in marriage only the duties it imposes; and they regard it only as the founding act of a society, since this society-to-be is, in the sacrament, the object of the blessings of religion, and, in the civil contract, the object of the clauses ratified and guaranteed by the State.

Any commitment between intelligent and sensible beings who have the faculty to will and to act presumes freedom in the will and strength in the action. Thus where there is recognized constraint or proven impotence there is no marriage, because there is no commitment and no society can be born. These two obstacles to marriage are called *diriment impediments*, and all other ones refer to them.

Once the commitment is valid, there can be no reason to dissolve it, even for the non-arrival of children.

The motives for indissolubility are taken from both domestic and public society, because marriage is both domestic in its principle and public in its effects.

1. Marriage is a *potential* society, the family an *actual* society. Nature has not set a term on this potential; and even when marriage does not attain its social goal, and children do not arrive, there is not a sufficient reason to break the first commitment in order to form another, because the fertility of

the second marriage is just as speculative as that of the first. Once the child has arrived, the goal is fulfilled, and the society, from being potential, becomes actual.

Thus, as long as the husband and wife have no children, they could still arrive; and since marriage is formed only for the children who are to come, there is no reason to break the marriage. Once the children have arrived, the marriage has attained its goal, and there is a reason not to break the marriage; for it is to be noted that impotence is not proved against the wife, even in the case of infertility.

In a word, the reason for marriage is the production of children. Now, by breaking a first marriage in order to contract a second one, this production becomes impossible in the first without becoming more certain in the second. Therefore, there is no reason to break the marriage; and after all, whatever disposition our modern philosophers may have to assimilate man to the beasts, and whatever importance may be attached to population by these great depopulators of the universe, they would doubtless not dare to maintain that in human marriages one should, as on stud farms, proceed by *trials*.

2. The reasons against divorce drawn from public society are even stronger than those taken from domestic society.

Political power cannot guarantee the stability of the domestic persons without knowing them; hence the necessity of the civil act, which makes known the commitment of the man and woman, and of the birth certificate, which makes known the father, mother, and child.

But, and I beg the reader to pay attention to this reasoning, political power only intervenes in the spouses' contract of union because it represents the unborn child, which is the sole social object of marriage, and because it accepts the commitment made by the spouses in its presence and under its guarantee to bring that child into being. It stipulates the interests of the child in the contract, since most matrimonial clauses concern the arrival of children, and since on occasion it even accepts certain special advantages, stipulated in advance, in favor of a child born in a certain order of birth or sex; and as witness of the bond which is to give the child existence, it guarantees the bond's stability in order to ensure the child's conservation. The marital commitment is thus really formed between three persons who are either present or represented; for public power, which precedes the family and survives it, always represents the absent person in the family, whether the child before its birth, or the father after his death.

The commitment formed between three therefore cannot be broken by two to the prejudice of the third, since this third person is, if not the first, at least the most important; since everything relates to him alone; and since he is the *reason* for the social union of the other two, who are no more a father or mother without the child than he is a son without them. "In ordinary societies," say the authors of the proposed Civil Code, "one stipulates for oneself; in marriage, one stipulates for another." A father and mother who divorce are thus really two strong people who conspire to rob a weak one, and the State which consents to this is an accomplice in their brigandage. This third person can never, even when present, consent to the dissolution of the society which gave him being, since he is always a *minor* in the family, even when he has reached his majority in the State, and consequently is always incapable of consenting to anything to his prejudice; and political power, which represented him in order to establish the bond of the society, can no longer represent him in order to dissolve it, because the tutor is given to the pupil less to accept what is to his benefit than to prevent what is to his detriment; which is why he can validly buy in his pupil's name but cannot sell in it.

Marriage is therefore indissoluble in terms of the domestic and public states of society. It is therefore naturally indissoluble: for the natural or man's nature is made up both of the domestic and public states; and there are certainly grounds for astonishment to hear the authors of the proposed Civil Code say that *marriage is neither a civil nor a religious act, but a natural one;* for if by a natural act they mean a physical act, then marriage is nothing but a meeting of animals; and if they mean something else, then it is impossible to guess what they wish to say.

Divorce is therefore contrary to the principle of society; we shall show, in the subsequent parts of this treatise, that it is destructive in its effects on society.

CHAPTER 5

Of the Three States of Society:
Imperfect; Perfect or Natural; Corrupted
or against Nature

THE organized beings which have an end and the external means to attain it are born in a state of weakness of means which prevents them from attaining their end. So begin man and society. This is the imperfect state; and it is imperfect since it tends toward another state which is better and stronger, and since the being perishes if it does not attain this latter state.

Time and acquisitions develop its means, and cause the being successively to pass to a more advanced state. Thus the seed becomes a plant, the fetus becomes a man, and a savage people becomes civilized.

Some use their developed means in the manner best suited to the end for which they exist, and attain that state which is called maturity in the plant, manhood and reason in man, and civilization in society. This is the perfect or natural state of beings. Others fall into an evil state, either because their means are insufficiently developed, because they have deviated in the course of their development, or because they do not use them in a manner appropriate to their end. For man, this is the state of bodily infirmity or moral weakness, either one of which makes man an overgrown child, or the state of bodily strength and disordered will, which makes him wicked or a *robust child,* as Hobbes calls him; in society, it is the state opposed to civilization. This state is evil, corrupt, unnatural.

Perfect or natural state; evil or unnatural state. We shall return to these shortly.

The individual man, to attain his individual conservation, which is his end, has a will and physical organs, the ministers or means of his will in the execution of his individual actions.

Society, to attain its end, which is its conservation, has laws, which are its will, and persons, the means or ministers of the laws in the execution of social action.

In the state of infancy or imperfection, man's will is as weak as his means; sometimes he uses much force to accomplish little, sometimes he tries to accomplish much with little force.

The wicked or insane man has a weak or disordered will served by powerful means; he destroys other beings, he destroys himself: this is the corrupt and evil state.

The perfected or good man has an enlightened will, and his will rules his actions. *The law of the members does not rebel against that of the mind,* and the body is obedient to reason, as the minister to the power, and the means to the cause.

Nascent society is in the imperfect state: it has weak laws and a weak or violent action, for violence is weakness; in the family, it is repudiation or polygamy, veritable domestic despotism; in the State, it is political despotism, which "subjects everything to its will and whims," says Montesquieu. Sometimes it acts without ministers, like Clovis, who personally split the skull of one of his soldiers, or Peter I, who personally decimated his streltsy; sometimes power is usurped by its ministers: by the mayors of the palace, under the kings of the first dynasty; by the bishops, under Louis the Debonair; by the patricians, as in Poland.

Corrupt society has a disordered will, or laws against nature, and a disordered action. In the family, it is divorce, which deposes the father and tears his children from him; it is infanticide, by which children perish at the father's hands; it is abominable loves; in the State, it is the people declaring itself sovereign. "The people in this state," the *Spirit of the Laws* says very well,[1] "always has too much or too little action; sometimes with a hundred thousand arms it overturns everything, sometimes with a hundred thousand feet it only moves like an insect." This people destroys other peoples and ends by destroying itself: "for if it wishes to harm itself," says the *Social Contract,* "who has the right to prevent it from doing so?" By these features one recognizes democracy, and it is Montesquieu and Rousseau who have named it.

In the good or perfect state of society, will, represented by the laws, is perfect, and action is ruled by will. Power is absolute and not arbitrary; the ministers are subordinate, the subjects obedient. This state of society rests on laws rather than persons; and the weak Louis XIII, when he had Montmorency condemned to death, denying his mercy to the tears of all France, possessed a power less arbitrary and more absolute than the strong Clovis, when, at Soissons, he personally administered justice to one of his soldiers.

These three states of society are clearly distinguished in religious society. The act of worship or the sacrifice was imperfect in the Judaic religion, and the beast was immolated to ransom the man.

In the Christian religion, the act or sacrifice is perfect, because, according to Christians, the victim is the most perfect of beings, and because, according to history, Christian society is the most enlightened and consequently the strongest of societies.

In the pagan religion, which was an evil and unnatural state of society, man himself was immolated to Divinity, and the gods themselves were nothing but corruption and license.

Thus, to enslave one's prisoner of war, to kill him, and to

---

[1] Charles-Louis de Secondat, baron de la Brède et de Montesquieu, *De l'esprit des loix,* 2 vols. (Geneva: Barillot et fils, 1748; many subsequent editions).

free him mark the distinction between the imperfect, corrupt, and perfect states of the law of nations among Christians and non-Christian peoples.

The perfection of the domestic and public laws is called civilization.

Thus civilization is the perfection of laws and morals, as refinement is the perfection of arts and manners; for manners are an art and morals a law.

Thus the Greeks, who had such clever sculptors, such fluent sages, such polished courtesans, but whose laws allowed prostitution to women, the killing of children, the murder of slaves, and abominable loves, were refined without being civilized; while the Germans, with their crude arts and natural manners, as Tacitus describes them, had a beginning of civilization, without refinement.

The perfect state of a being is its natural state, because a being's natural state is that in which its being is completed, fulfilled; and because properly speaking it *is* not, so long as it has not attained that state, and ceases to be if it does not attain it.

Thus the natural or perfect state of the seed is to become a plant, of the fetus to become a man, of the savage people to become civilized; and the seed, the fetus, and the people perish if they do not in some sense attain this perfect state.

The imperfect state of a being is thus not its natural state but its native or *original* state, and this distinction is fundamental.

Thus nature in general is the totality of the perfect laws of beings, as the particular nature of a being is the totality of its particular laws; and it is an absurdity to have made nature the legislator of the universe, when it is only the legislation.

This is modern philosophy's great quarrel with reason. Jean-Jacques Rousseau locates the natural state of individual or social man in the native or imperfect state. This is the source of his predilection for children, at least for those of other people, and of his mindless admiration for the savage state.

Hence these propositions worthy of the madhouse: "The man who thinks is a depraved animal"; "man is born good, and society depraves him."

Thus a being's imperfect state is a native or original state, but the perfect or natural state is an acquired or adventitious state, from *adventitius,* which means *of external origin.*

"Certain philosophers," says very well the great Leibniz, "locate nature in the state which has the least art, failing to notice that *perfection* always includes art."

Thus the adult is more natural than the child, the educated man more natural than the ignorant one, the virtuous man more natural than the vicious one, and the civilized man more natural than the savage. That is why nothing is harder to acquire than naturalness in works of the mind; and why, in laws as in art, in morals as in manners, the false, the bad, the *unnatural* presents itself to our minds of its own accord. *Verum,* says Quintilian, *id est maxime quod natura fieri optime patitur:*[2] thus recognizing that the natural state is both an acquired and a perfect state, *fieri optime.*[3]

Thus reason also locates the imperfect state in the original or native state.

Nature and art are thus not opposed to each other, and this figure of speech, transported into legislation, has produced deplorable errors.

It was thought that there were *natural* laws, as there are *natural* needs; and Jean-Jacques Rousseau went so far as to say, "What God wills man to do, he does not tell him through another man, he tells it to him himself, and writes it at the bottom of his heart"; and it was not seen that if even the most natural of laws were natural in this sense, then man could no more disregard the laws of society than the laws of digestion. From this idea of *natural laws written by God himself at the*

[2] "The true is above all that which nature allows to be done in the best way." This passage has not been found in Quintilian.
[3] "To be done in the best way."

bottom of our hearts followed the idea of artificial laws, written by men on marble and brass, which were called *positive,* and the latter were considered to be less obligatory than the former. Thus, *honor your father* was a *natural* law, and *honor the political power* a *positive* law; and often one vaunted the natural virtues of men or sects that disregarded their public duties, and that in marriage, for instance, made an infidelity a crime, and divorce a duty or at least a good deed.

In another regard, as the religion of primitive families was exclusively called *natural,* and the religion of the State was exclusively called *revealed,* it was concluded that only primitive or patriarchal religion was natural, and that the religion of the State was *artificial, and the religion of priests.*

Let us dare, then, if not to reform, at least to clarify this equivocal language, and say, that *natural* or domestic religion was natural to the man of the primitive family, considered before the emergence of any public state of society, and that revealed or public religion is natural to the man of the family considered in the public state. Let us say, that domestic religion was revealed by speech, and public religion was revealed by writing; because everything man knows of his duties, even his religious ones, comes to him through revelation, that is to say, through speech which conveys to him the expression of his own ideas. This is the sublime doctrine of Saint Paul, veritable apostle of nations, because he taught the science of society. He says, like Jean-Jacques Rousseau, that we carry a law written at the bottom of our hearts, *lex scripta in cordibus nostris;*[4] but far from saying, "What God wills man to do, he does not tell him through another man," Saint Paul expressly states that "knowledge comes from hearing; and man cannot hear unless he is spoken to": *Fides ex auditu; quomodo audient sine praedicante?*[5] Which means that we have in our-

---

[4] "The law is written in our hearts." Paul, Romans 2.15.
[5] "Faith comes from hearing . . . how shall they hear without a preacher?" Paul, Romans 10.17, 10.14.

selves, as natural, the knowledge necessary for our happiness; but to be perceptible by our minds, it must be clothed in expressions, as bodies, to be visible, need light sensible by our eyes; an essential difference from the beasts, which also hear speech, and sometimes repeat it, but do not associate it with any idea, because they have no ideas, and have at most only images.

Let us say, that positive or political legislation is as natural as so-called *natural* legislation, because the State is as natural to the conservation of families as the family itself is to the propagation of man; and that nowhere has one ever seen man born without a family, or families conserving themselves without forming a public State. Let us say, that laws are not natural because *God has written them at the bottom of our hearts;* nor artificial because they are promulgated by man; but that domestic or public laws are natural when they are perfect or in conformity with the natural relationships of beings, and that all good, perfect, and natural laws given to men emanate from God as the supreme reason and general will, and are proclaimed by a man as the voice of his will and the means of their transmission to man.

So therefore, if one were to write a treatise of general legislation,* instead of following these obscure and equivocal definitions of natural and positive laws, and natural and positive rights, one would divide the laws into domestic and public laws; into religious and political laws; into good or natural laws, and bad or unnatural ones; and one would say with Cicero that "the rule which serves to distinguish a good law from a bad is found only in nature," *legem bonam a mala, nulla alia nisi* naturali *norma, dividere possumus.*[6]

Natural laws are those of the *beginning*, since the relationships between beings which they express are as old as the

---

*That is what the author has tried to do in the *First Laws.*
[6]Cicero, *On the Laws* 1.16.44.

beings themselves; they are also laws of the *end,* since beings can only attain their end by conforming themselves to it; they are the *alpha* and *omega* of beings; and it is in this sense that Jesus Christ calls the law of marital indissolubility "the law of the beginning": *Ab initio non fuit sic.*[7]

A society can no more remain in the imperfect state than man can remain in childhood. Both always advance toward *consummation,* and the only stationary state is the finished, perfect or natural state.

Reason conceives that a people may pass from the imperfect state to the perfect state; this is the law of nature and the march of beings. The law of repudiation, permitted to the Jews, gave way to Christian indissolubility, and their sacrifice to that of the Christians. Thus in France, arbitrary power under Clovis became absolute under Philip Augustus. This theory of the imperfect or legal state which precedes the perfect state, and which, weak and useless for society's end, is rejected and transformed into a better state, is admirably expounded in Saint Paul's Epistles to the Romans and the Hebrews. *Nihil enim,* he says, *ad perfectum adducit lex . . . reprobatio quidem fit praecedentis mandati, propter infirmitatem ejus et inutilitatem.*[8]

If the imperfect state does not attain the perfect state, it transforms itself into the evil state. The Greeks and even the Romans passed from the despotism of their first kings to popular government, and from repudiation to divorce, as their ancestors had passed from natural religion to idolatry. But a society which cannot, without perishing, remain in the imperfect state, can still less remain in the evil state opposed to its natural end, the object of the constant tendency of all beings. "For," Jean-Jacques Rousseau says very well, "if the legis-

[7] "It was not so from the beginning." Matthew 19.8.
[8] "For the law brings nothing to perfection. . . . Indeed it is a rejection of the earlier command, on account of its weakness and uselessness." Hebrews 7.19, 7.18.

lator, mistaking his object, establishes a principle different from that which arises from the nature of things, the State (*society*) will not cease to be agitated until it is destroyed or changed, and invincible nature has resumed her sway."

Thus the Jews could not remain under the imperfect state of their religion without continually falling into the last excesses of idolatry. Toward the end of their existence as a national body, the sect of the Pharisees had altered the worship with their traditions, and that of the Sadducees had ruined the dogma with their opinions; and what is truly marvelous in this people is to see it today with a religion without ministers, and a form of worship without sacrifice—this people whose worship was nothing but sacrifices, and whose ministers made up such a large part of the nation—remaining stationary in this more than imperfect state, and, while rejecting Christianity, preserving itself equally from atheism and idolatry: an extraordinary state, even a supernatural one in the eyes of an enlightened reason, since it is opposed to nature or the laws of beings in society.

The passage from the imperfect to the perfect state of society is practicable, since it has been practiced; and it is natural to man, since the Northern peoples, from whom modern peoples are descended, all passed from the imperfect and crude state of their natural religion, and of their polygamous or despotic society, to Christianity, monogamy, and monarchy.

But when once a nation has attained the perfect state, *and has tasted the heavenly gift of natural laws,* it cannot descend from thence without falling into the last degree of misery and degradation, because this retrograde journey is contrary to all the laws of the nature of beings and all the perceptions of reason. Thus Poland, having fallen, upon the extinction of the Jagiellon dynasty, into the imperfect state of political society, and soon after into that of religious and even of domestic society as well, was, after three centuries of torpor and convulsions, *at least for a time,* erased from the rank of nations.

France, having fallen into the monarchical democracy of 1789, descended to the vile and bloody demagogy of 1793; and who would dare to contemplate the probable consequences of this revolutionary delirium, if the principle of life which fourteen centuries of constitution had given this society had not drawn it from the abyss of shame, corruption, and sorrow.

Thus a nation declines and falls when it descends from the perfect state; and a nation merely vegetates and languishes as long as it is unable to attain that state; as witness the Oriental peoples, Turks, Chinese, Persians, Indians, the weakest of all peoples; for as to the true Tartar, he is the strongest of all non-Christian peoples, because his political constitution is natural, his religion rather imperfect than corrupt, and because in his case refinement did not precede civilization; a people which is always young, as long as it is not established and lives under its tents, where all nations begin and begin anew, even those which have ended in the boudoirs and at the theaters.

There is thus no rest for a people but in society's perfect state; there alone is its true strength, because strength is in stability, and stability can only be found in the finished state; and although no society is in this fulfilled state, no more than any man, one can observe, in the social world, more enlightenment, virtue, strength, and resolve among the Christians than among other peoples, and even in Europe, more disinterestedness, greatness, and sobriety, more progress in the arts of knowledge, more real strength, finally, and resolve, among certain peoples than others.

The passage from the imperfect state to the perfect state takes place without effort, because it is natural. Christianity, an object of persecution in the Roman empire, caused no troubles in it. The conversion of the Franks did not lead to civil war. That of several thousand Chinese has produced none in China. But the return from a better to a worse state cannot take place without difficulty and pain, because it is contrary to the law of nature.

There, and there alone, is the true reason for the rise and decadence of nations. The vicissitude of human affairs, on which commonplaces have been lavished for so many centuries, is a true idea, no doubt, if understood in terms of the natural and necessary tendency of all created beings to attain that natural order to which they aspire, and in which alone they can find rest; *omnis creatura ingemiscit;*[9] but a false and even impious idea if understood in terms of a blind and inevitable necessity of change, *ferrea necessitas,*[10] which is sometimes offered as a consolation to those whom one has reduced to misery: as if any event, under the law of the supreme reason, could be subject to no law, and have no reason; and as if instability could be necessary in the creature, when the will of the creator is immutable.

The Assyrians, Medes, Romans, and Greeks perished because they had passed from the imperfect state of nascent peoples to the corrupt state of degenerate peoples. The Northern peoples continue to exist in Europe, stronger than at the time of their establishment, because they have passed from the imperfect to the perfect state of society; and among the Turks, the most extreme weakness only succeeded to that access of delirium which for a moment made them the terror of Christianity because they were unable to escape the imperfect state of polygamy, despotism, and deism.

These great lessons of history are surely better understood today: France has in a sense summarized them, in the latest experiment she has performed on herself; and it would be terrible for a nation to perish when it has, *by eating the forbidden fruit,* acquired the science of good and evil, so that the choice between them lies in the hands of those who govern it.

The principles of the two societies, domestic and public, are similar: the effects will be similar in both. We have sought the

[9] "The whole creation groans." Paul, Romans 8.22.
[10] "Iron necessity."

principles in the constitution of societies; next we shall observe the effects in their history. It is inseparably connected
with that of divorce, and should throw the greatest light on that
question.

CHAPTER 6

Of Society among the Jews

THE plurality of unions or polygamy*—whether potential, through the faculty of repudiation, as among the Jews, or actual, through cohabitation, as among the Turks—can be tolerated for families in that purely domestic state of society which precedes any public establishment and is called the *patriarchal state,* or when, having recently left that state, families retain its habits; because the multiplication of the species, which polygamy encourages at this age of society alone, may be appropriate to a small tribe which is trying to raise itself to the strength and dignity of a nation.

This law is not contrary to physical nature, since it does not prevent the reproduction of beings, and several children can be born to a single father and several mothers; but it is imperfect in moral terms, because it breaks moral unity or the union of hearts, by placing several societies in a single family, and several interests in a single household.

Yet polygamy, which is merely imperfect in society's nascent state, becomes evil in its advanced state, because at this age of a nation, communication between the sexes—having become more frequent through the proximity of families, and less innocent through the taste for pleasure and the progress of the arts, which follows that of wealth—inflames the passion of love; a passion without danger among a nascent people, because it follows the union of the sexes there; but a terrible

*Polygamy, monogamy do not signify plurality, unity of women, although usage gives them this acceptation, but plurality or unity of marriage; and in this sense, a woman can be polygamous.

passion when it precedes that union, as among an advanced
people, where it transforms the faculty of repudiation into a
traffic in adulteresses, and polygamy into a barbarous jail
where men are mutilated to watch over women; a state which
is then contrary to the being's nature, even its physical one,
and which produces the oppression of humanity, the neglect of
children, and even, as the author of the *Spirit of the Laws*
observes, unnatural loves, of which he cites some remarkable
examples; a state which is consequently opposed to nature;
and the Turks are only perishing because, in the state of
nationhood, they persist in retaining a law which is only bear-
able in the state of the family, considered before the existence
of any nation.

In this original or nearly original state of society, since
population is a necessity, sterility is a curse; it is even a
disgrace, and whatever may alter the union is a crime. The
husband dismisses his wife for sterility, and even for not being
found pleasing, *propter foeditatem.*[1] This is the law of the
Jews,* a law clearly directed wholly toward the multiplication
of the people, a law which is consequently appropriate to the
infancy of a nation; and what demonstrates this is that still
today, among savages, as formerly among the Jews, a brother
marries his brother's widow, and for the same reason. Let us
pause for a moment over the law of repudiation, which the
innovators have used to authorize establishing divorce.

The law which allows repudiation is an imperfect one, which
considers marriage more as a proximity of bodies than as a
bond of hearts, since it dissolves marriage for bodily infir-

---

*The law of Moses condemns an adulterous woman to death. It was an act of
humanity on the part of the husband to restrict himself to repudiation when
he could have required her execution. M. l'abbé Bergier, who offers this
reflection, assumes that, then as now, the law did not punish a guilty person
twice for the same crime. *Non bis in idem.*[2]
[1] "On account of ugliness."
[2] "Not twice for the same thing."

mities. It is even a harsh law, since it punishes a woman for the offenses of nature; takes away her social existence, in the uncertain hope of a more fertile union; and, finally, because it lays on her alone the misfortune of a sterile union, whose fault could also be imputed to her spouse, and is in fact never proved against the wife.

But this law is not contrary to the nature of beings in society, that is to say, it is not destructive of the natural relationships of power and its subordinates, since it leaves exclusively in the man the essential attribute of power, the right to contest and judge the actions of the woman, and since it does not separate the children from their father. This power vested in the man is even excessive, and carried to the point of despotism; and here one can observe that at the birth of domestic society, as at that of public society, power is always less regulated and more violent.

One therefore sees the motive for repudiation among the Jews—an imperfect law, and which *was only for a time, like everything imperfect,* but which was not evil or contrary to nature—and one is even led to believe, as many interpreters have maintained, that repudiation among the Jews was only a separation *a mensa et a toro,*[3] which allowed the man, but not the woman, to contract another union, since the law of *Deuteronomy* calls the dismissed wife who has passed to a second marriage *soiled and abominable before the Lord.* Josephus expressly states, book 15, chapter 11, that the laws do not allow repudiated wives to remarry without the consent of their husbands. But this discussion is of no interest here.

Among a nascent people, the law of repudiation, which is purely optional, has no dangerous consequences, because it is seldom used. When the family lives a rural life, isolated from other families, occupied with healthier work, and nourished with more wholesome food, there are fewer of those desires in

[3] "From bed and board."

the sexes which provoke repudiation, and fewer of the infirmities which justify it. At this age of society, man's dominant
passion is not voluptuousness, and the husband considers his
wife more in terms of the services he extracts from her than in
terms of her external charms. This observation can be verified
by our eyes in the lower classes, where the people are always
at the earliest age of society. In general, the more a people
lives in the domestic state, the more the women are dependent
and even subservient. The savage leaves all unpleasant tasks to
his wife. The same was true among the Germans; and still
today, in some of France's southern provinces, subject to
Roman law, where the relationships of the domestic persons
are more strongly marked, the same peasant who regards
divorce only with horror would think himself lacking toward a
stranger whom he honors and receives in his house, if he
seated his wife at the same table.

But in proportion as Judaic society passed from the domestic to the public state, the law of repudiation suited it less,
because it was used more often. Little by little this condescension of the legislator produced a frenzied libertinism. "One
reads in the *Synopsis of the Critics*," says the abbé de Rastignac, "that Naaman had a herald proclaim: *What woman will I
have each day, or during my sojourn here?*"[4] The school of the
rabbi *Hillel* taught that a man could repudiate his wife for
having burned the soup; and the rabbi *Akiba*, who had as
many as eighty thousand followers, taught that a husband
could dismiss his wife solely because he found another more
beautiful, or even without any pretext at all. But in the family
as in the State, the abuse of power prepares its fall: the excess
of repudiation brought on reciprocal divorce; the law gave the

[4] Matthew Poole, *Synopsis criticorum aliorumque Sacrae Scripturae inter-
pretum et commentatorum,* 3 vols. (London: Flesher, 1669–1673; new editions in 1680 and 1684–1686), vol. 3. Cited in the abbé Armand de Chapt de
Rastignac's *Accord de la Révélation et de la Raison contre le divorce* (Paris:
Clousier, 1790), p. 100.

husband the power to repudiate his wife, the wife usurped, in the end, the power to repudiate her husband,* and the first example of this was given by Salome, the sister of Herod the Great, "who," says Josephus, bk. 15, "sent a notice of repudiation to her husband Costobarus, an Idumaean, contrary to the custom of our laws, which assign this power to husbands alone."

The government of the family among the Jews was thus severe to the point of harshness: and note too that the government of this people by God himself was extremely severe as well, and that it was only by blood-soaked executions, and by delivering it up to all the scourges, that he held this constantly rebellious slave to the path of duty.

Mosaic law consecrated paternal power no less than it did marital authority. This law—often imperfect but always natural—by giving the father of the family an absolute authority over his children, forestalled the danger of an arbitrary use of authority, which it strengthened both by the rights it attributed to the father and by those it reserved to public power. Thus, it gave the father of the family the power to repudiate his wife, and the more terrible power to disinherit an ungrateful child from the paternal blessing. But wiser than the pagan laws, this law, which prohibited cooking a goat in its mother's milk, took care not to allow the father to shed his son's blood; and it reserved to public power the right to execute the adulterous wife and the rebellious child. The natural relationships between the domestic persons were therefore conserved by Mosaic law; morals, which are the domestic laws, were therefore good among this people, and are still good today, when the morals of Jewish families are no longer under the protection of their laws.

I have intentionally insisted on the difference between repudiation and mutual divorce, and between an imperfect law

---

*Jesus Christ rebuked the Samaritan woman for having had five husbands.

and a vicious and unnatural one, because this essential, fundamental difference has not been sufficiently felt. Repudiation conserves the husband's natural power to judge the wife and condemn her to dismissal; and *it is always an act of jurisdiction, even when it is not an act of justice*. Reciprocal divorce gives the wife jurisdiction over the husband, by attributing to her the power to judge and condemn him, whether she herself provokes the divorce or whether she merely ratifies it. Thus, because the woman is weaker, she uses this usurped power more often. Divorce is provoked by wives more often than by husbands; and, according to Mme. Necker, "the confederacy of women who solicit divorce is very numerous." M. de Montesquieu sensed the difference between repudiation and divorce; but what he says of it here is no more accurate than what he has written elsewhere on this matter. "There is," he says, "this difference between divorce and repudiation: divorce takes place by mutual consent, in the event of a mutual incompatibility, whereas repudiation takes place at the will of one of the parties, independently of the will and interest of the other." This definition, in which the author presumes there are two wills in the family, and consequently two powers in it, is inexact, since divorce can be obtained, and very often is, without the consent and even despite the opposition of one of the parties, which finds no incompatibility in living with the other party, and often even when it places its happiness or at least its duty in enduring the other one.

It must be concluded, from the real difference we have just established between repudiation and mutual divorce, and from the natural reason on which it is based, that God, who tolerated an imperfect law among the Jews, would not have allowed them an unnatural one, like a father who closes his eyes to a child's pranks, but punishes its disobedience.

CHAPTER 7

Of Society among the Orientals, Greeks, and Romans

THE simultaneous plurality of women was accepted among the Asiatics, as it still is today, for this childish people has never been able to escape the imperfect state. But as I have already observed, this form of marriage carries to excess the husband's power and the wife's dependence. This domestic despotism therefore accords with political despotism, and political despotism in turn maintains and strengthens domestic despotism. Such has been the case at all times in the Orient; such is still the case there, and there have always been slaves in the family and slaves in the State. Children in Egypt do not dare to sit in front of their elders, while the people tremble in front of the beys; and it is only the excess of domestic power which, in that unhappy country, as formerly in Rome, maintains families in some form of public state of society.

Whether the mutual faculty of divorce was the cause of popular government or its effect, it is certain that mutual divorce, veritable domestic democracy, which gives the weak party in society jurisdiction over the strong one, and even the right to depose it, in order to convey the power elsewhere, is found among the Greeks alongside public or political democracy, which attributes sovereign power to the people, along with the faculty of delegating it: for the people, like woman, only divorces power to pass to a second commitment; and when God, in Scripture, rebukes the Jewish people for wishing to renounce his alliance, he never calls it anything but the *adulterous* people.

It was therefore in the Athenian democracy that the laws of

Solon, for the first time, allowed divorce to the wife, which she may have allowed to herself earlier than the law. This childish people, as Plato calls it in the *Timaeus,* among which, he says, there were never any old men, because it never advanced in social life; this people, in its vain wisdom, which it always sought outside of nature, *Graeci sapientiam quaerunt,*[1] denatured all things in domestic, political, and religious society. It brought the law of mutual divorce into the family, and that of abominable loves: *Mihi quidem haec in Graecorum gymnasiis nata consuetudo videtur, in quibus isti liberi et concessi sunt amores,* says Cicero.[2] It taught the Universe atheism:

> *Primum Graius homo mortales tollere contra*
> *Est oculos ausus*

says Lucretius.[3] It caused political power to pass into the hands of the people, and abolished the unity of power, because of the virtues of Codrus; considerably less reasonable in this regard than the Romans, who at least sought a pretext in the vices of Tarquin. Finally, with its arts and its letters, it lost everything in morals and laws, as Cato the Elder reproached it for having done: *Gens ista quoties litteras suas dabit, omnia perdet.*[4]

As one advances in the world's history, one often finds the same domestic, political, and religious disorders together: for everything denatures itself at the same time in man.

Thus, in the Italian democracies of the Middle Ages, the abominable morals of the Greeks were visible alongside the turbulence of their political institutions. Thus, philosophy

[1] "The Greeks seek wisdom." Paul, 1 Corinthians 1.22.
[2] "To me at least this custom seems to have been born in the gymnasia of the Greeks, where that sort of love affair is free and permitted." Cicero, *Tusculan Disputations* 4.33.70.
[3] "It was a Greek who first dared to lift mortal eyes against [religion]." Lucretius, *On the Nature of Things* 1.66–67.
[4] "When that race gives us its letters, it will destroy everything." Cato the Censor, *Fragments of Letters to His Son Marcus,* fragment 1 = Pliny, *Natural History* 29.14.

could not rouse the peoples against their heads without rousing wives and children against husbands and fathers, men against God, and even without authorizing the most monstrous disorders; and the proof of this is visible in Condorcet's posthumous work. "Therefore," says the proposed Civil Code, "one overthrows the power of fathers, because children are more susceptible to novelties; marital authority is not respected, because it is by giving women greater freedom that one manages to introduce new forms and a new tone."

But men stray from nature, and cannot destroy it: even among the Greeks, the terms in which divorce was expressed and the forms required to obtain it conserved some traces of the natural superiority of the husband and the natural dependence of the wife, of the power of the former to repudiate, and of the crime committed by the latter in breaking the conjugal tie with her own hands. When divorce was requested by the husband, it was called *dismissal,* when requested by the wife, *abandonment;* and the law, which subjected a wife who provoked a divorce to the humiliating ceremony of presenting her request in person to the magistrate, did not impose the same requirement on the husband. What shows the close association of mutual divorce and democracy is that divorce was only practiced among the Athenians, and that in Sparta, where the people had no part of power, wives were not allowed to leave their husbands. No law in the code of Lycurgus authorizes mutual divorce. The Greeks, in the heroic and monarchical ages, were unfamiliar with it. *Gronovius* concludes this, and rightly so, from a passage in Euripides' *Medea;** and the Trojan War would have been pointless if, by

---

Non enim honesta sunt divortia mulieribus, neque licet mulieri abdicare maritum (Euripid. Medea, l. 230).[5] The expression *abdicare* is remarkable: as if a woman who divorces really abdicates power over herself, and becomes the slave of her passions.

[5] "Divorce is discreditable to women, nor is a woman allowed to repudiate [literally, abdicate] her husband." A loose translation of Euripides, *Medea* 236–237.

the favor of a divorce, Helen could have abandoned her first husband to join her new lover.

Among the Greeks as everywhere, paternal power followed the fortunes of marital power; it was of no account in Athens, and all the stronger in Sparta in that every child was reputed to have as many fathers as there were old men. Thus in both cities domestic power, which is composed of marital and paternal authority, was constituted like public power: opposite constitutions, which produced the most turbulent, frivolous, weak, and sometimes cruel people in Greece, and the gravest, wisest, and strongest.

In Rome, the family began by repudiation, as the State began by despotism; for, as M. de Montesquieu observes very well, none of the ancient States was founded *on any fundamental law*. But when, through the violence of the last kings, or rather through the ambition of a number of senators, the State had fallen into the government of several, or aristocracy, while waiting to fall into the government of all, or demagogic anarchy, the sword, essential attribute of society's conservative power, passed to or remained in the family; and a law of Valerius Publicola even took away the magistrate's power to condemn citizens to death. The father had the right of life and death over his son, the husband over his wife, the master over his slaves, and even on occasion, in time of civil troubles, the citizen over the citizen. Domestic power even wielded the atrocious right to take the life of the child: for it was not enough for the child that the father had given it life, but paternal power had to permit the child to enjoy it as well. At birth, the child was placed at the feet of the despot, who, by raising it from the ground, allowed it to live (this is the source of our expression *to raise a child*); and the father could condemn an innocent child to death, at a time when the magistrate could only sentence a guilty subject to exile.

The weakness of the first Romans, their rural life, and this terrible power of the father of the family, maintained for a time their private morals against laws which were either bad or imperfect. For several centuries, indeed, repudiation was unknown in their midst, because all the pretexts for dismissal, and even all its grounds, are rarer among a simple agricultural people. But in proportion as the nation grew and developed, the inadequacy of this imperfect constitution of domestic and public power made itself felt, and at almost the same time, in both family and State. The same secular revolution (for centuries are the years of society) witnessed both the dissolution of the conjugal tie, through the example given by Carvilius Ruga, who repudiated his wife in the year 523 of the founding of Rome, and the dissolution of the State, through the passage from aristocracy to demagogy under the Gracchi around 620, or even earlier, through the establishment of the power of the decemvirs and tribunes; *non populi sed plebis magistratus,* says Livy.[6] The degeneration increased steadily in one society as in the other, because power lay nowhere; the level of corruption became monstrous, as the level of austerity had been excessive. The husband had repudiated the wife; now the wife dismissed her husband, and counted her years, as Seneca says, not by the names of the consuls but by the number of her husbands. The father had caused the death of his son; the son in turn caused the death of his father, by denouncing him in the proscriptions. Disorder never ceased again in Rome, and to the last days of the empire there was license in the family and violence in the State.*

Uncertainty reigns among ancient authors as to whether the transition from repudiation to mutual divorce, from the imperfect state to the corrupted state, took place in Rome through morals or through laws. It appears from a passage in Plautus, in his comedy of the *Merchant,* that around the year 563 of

---

*Juvenal turns his satiric verve on the ladies of Rome, who discovered the means to change husbands eight times in five years. Saint Jerome recounts that he saw a woman buried in Rome who had had twenty-two husbands.
[6] "Magistrates not of the people but of the plebeians." Livy 2.56.12.

Rome, the right to repudiate had not yet been accorded to
the wife. Plutarch claims that Domitian was the first to allow
divorce to women. Others move the institution of this law up
to Julian the Apostate, which is to say, well after divorce had
been practiced. M. de Montesquieu thinks on the contrary,
after Cicero, that "the law ceaselessly corrupted morals"; and
I shall cite him here in support of everything I have said in this
chapter concerning Greek and Roman legislation relative to
marriage, and even on the difference between divorce and
repudiation.

> Romulus (he says) allowed the husband to repudiate his wife
> if she had committed an adultery, prepared poison, or counter-
> feited the keys. He did not give wives the right to repudiate their
> husbands. Plutarch calls this law, a very harsh law.
> As the law of Athens gave the wife, as well as the husband,
> the faculty of repudiation; and as one sees that wives obtained
> this right among the earliest Romans, notwithstanding the law
> of Romulus, it is clear that this institution was one of those
> which the deputies of Rome brought back from Athens, and
> that it was placed among the laws of the Twelve Tables.
> Cicero says that the grounds for repudiation came from the
> law of the Twelve Tables. . . . The faculty of divorce was more-
> over a provision, or at least a consequence, of the law of the
> Twelve Tables. For from the moment that the wife and the
> husband possessed separately the right of repudiation, there
> was all the more reason for them to be able to leave each other
> by mutual consent.
> The law did not require that one present any grounds for
> divorce. This is because, in the nature of the thing, grounds are
> required for repudiation, but not for divorce; since where the
> law establishes grounds for breaking marriage, mutual incom-
> patibility is the strongest of them all.

And concerning the act of Carvilius Ruga, which he disputes, although it is advanced by Dionysius of Halicarnassus,
Valerius Maximus, and Aulus Gellius, who credit the religion
of the auspices for the Romans' respect for the bonds of

marriage during the first centuries of the republic, M. de Montesquieu adds:

> The law of the Twelve Tables and the morals of the Romans greatly extended the law of Romulus. But if the citizens had so much respect for the auspices that they never engaged in repudiation, *why did the legislators of Rome have less respect than they? And how did the law ceaselessly corrupt morals?*

I shall further cite Mme. Necker on the same subject.[7]

> It was not divorce which was permitted in Rome, but repudiation only. In those centuries close to the state of nature, *the sexes were in no sense equal in rights,* strength reigned, and divorce would have been regarded as a law of dementia.
>
> In all times and places, women have been predisposed to safeguard morals; but the more sacred one considers the trust, the more one supervises and subjugates the trustee. Among the Romans, divorce was a punishment rather than a convention; they avenged themselves of their guilty wives in two equally dreaded ways, through actual death, or through repudiation, a kind of civil death, a death in opinion. . . . The Roman ladies, subject to such severe laws, gave their husbands little cause for complaint, and it should be no surprise that a hundred years passed without a single instance of repudiation. But what comparison is there between divorce as received among the Romans and as just adopted (in 1792)? One was a law of modesty, the other a law of audacity. In Rome divorce was the guardian of morals, in France it will be their corruptor; and if repudiation as authorized among the Romans had been admitted in our midst, women would have always been its victims. . . . Nevertheless, and despite the one-sidedness of a law which would give the freedom to divorce to men only, this form *would injure good morals less,* which, *in accordance with nature,* always give women the privilege of one virtue more.

But nature never loses her rights, and she is found in opinions even when she no longer exists in either morals or laws.

[7] Suzanne Curchod Necker, *Réflexions sur le divorce* (Lausanne: Durand Ravanel, 1794).

The Romans regarded the disruption of marriage as one of the
most potent causes of disorder:

> *Foecunda culpae saecula nuptias*
> *Primum inquinavere*

says Horace.[8]

On the funerary monuments raised to wives one reads, as
the highest possible praise of their virtues, that they had had
only one husband:

> *Conjugi piae, inclytae, univirae,* etc.[9]

Divorce was forbidden to the Flamines, according to a
number of authors; Valerius Maximus says that second marriages are a confession of intemperance; and the Roman laws
speak of such marriages in harsh and odious terms: *matre,*
they say, *jam secundis nuptiis funestata.*[10]

Polygamy, whether actual or, through repudiation and divorce, potential, was thus practiced among the Orientals,
Jews, Greeks, and Romans: among all peoples which passed
from the domestic to some public state of society; and along
with it there reigned, through the whole idolatrous universe,
the oppression of age, sex, and condition, infanticide, slavery,
divination, religious prostitution, blood-soaked spectacles,
human victims, etc., etc., and even among the Jews, an extreme penchant for superstition and idolatry.

The law of the Jews was only for a time, *like every imperfect*

---

[8] "Ages fertile in sin first stained marriage." Horace, *Odes* 3.6.17–18. This
quotation serves as an epigraph to Hubert de Matigny's *Traité philosophique, théologique et politique de la loi du divorce, demandé aux Etats-
Généraux par S.A.S. Mgr. Louis-Philippe-Joseph d'Orléans, premier Prince
du Sang* (June 1789). This work favors "limited divorce" *(le divorce limité).*
[9] "For a wife who was loyal, honorable, had only one husband," etc. A
common sentiment on Roman tombs.
[10] "A mother now disgraced by a second marriage."

law: for the time of the infancy of social man, until the appearance of the legislator of the age of manhood, able to form, as Saint Paul says, *virum perfectum in mensuram aetatis plenitudinis Christi.*[11] For whether or not one accepts the divinity of the legislation of Moses, one cannot help seeing in the books of the Jews the announcement of a better legislation, and in the universe the actual existence of better laws; and the Jews themselves always awaited another legislator, since they await him still.

The times were accomplished, and this legislator appeared to society.

[11] "A man perfect in the measure of the age of the fullness of Christ." Paul, Ephesians 4.13.

CHAPTER 8

Of Society among Christian Peoples

THE progress of human knowledge follows the march of the centuries, because human knowledge rests on the experience of the ages. The sages of Greece and Rome may have had more upright hearts than our sages, and some of them may have had more penetrating minds; but there was less enlightenment in their time than in ours, because the world had lived less, and man had less experience. If today, after five thousand years of Mosaic legislation, which the ancients did not know or only knew imperfectly; after two thousand years of Christianity, which they could not witness; fourteen centuries of religious and political constitutions in Europe, founded on natural laws; three centuries of the most learned political and religious discussion; finally, ten years of a politico-religious revolution, and an experiment which can be regarded as the digest of the entire history of human societies; if today the authors of the proposed new Civil Code, distinguished for their learning in a nation which is itself distinguished for its advances; after having recognized this truth unknown to the ancients: "when abuses are the work of the passions, they can be corrected by the laws; but when they are the work of the laws, *the evil is incurable, because it lies in the cure itself"*; if they have presented the law of divorce as a cure for the evil of separa- tion, and have thereby set, as they themselves say, "a regular libertinism and an authorized inconstancy in the place of marriage itself"; if they have laid down as a principle that "laws are made for men, and should never be more perfect than men's state admits of," instead of recognizing that laws are promulgated against men's passions, and should be as perfect today as society's age allows and its needs require; if, in the nineteenth century, when *everything is consummated* for society, they allow divorce to Frenchmen, while it is necessary to begin the education of the savage by forbidding him polygamy; if, finally, when there can only be a question of more or less perfect, but always natural laws, they give us a vicious and unnatural one, by allowing the wife to revolt against her husband and tear his children from him; then I say with deep conviction: the legislator of the Christians, had he been only a man, would have known no more of his time than the authors of the proposed Civil Code know of theirs, because they have added eighteen centuries of experience to that which he had in his time, and because the man who is ahead of other men is never ahead of society. He would therefore have thought and spoken as men of the past thought and spoke; he would have, like our legislators, *consulted morals and characters,* accommodated his laws to men's penchants, instead of rectifying their penchants by his laws; and far from stopping at divorce, which was no longer a cure for an evil but a means to commit it, he would have sought a cure for divorce itself; and as our legislators have only been able to correct the abuse of separations through divorce, he would only have corrected the abuse of divorce through the community of women, which he found recommended in the laws of Plato, and the example, or nearly so, in the morals of all peoples, including his own. If he had not made his laws *more perfect than the men of that time admitted of,* then what laws would he have given to men, to women, as they are depicted by Juvenal, Tacitus, Petronius, Suetonius, and Josephus, last historian of the Jews? If he had given men only the laws they could admit of, then men—if indeed the human species had been able to survive this ghastly legislation—would today be worse than their laws; and Europe, the center of all civilization and refinement, Europe, which has made the whole universe the tributary of her knowl-

edge and strength, and where there lies, so to speak, the
general depot of all truths and virtues, of everything natural in
laws and arts, Europe would, like the rest of the world, be
given over to every error and disorder. May eternal thanks be
given him! It is not thus that the legislator of the Christians
considers man and society. He knows man and his penchants,
because he knows his work and that of man; and far from
presenting man with weak laws, the accomplices of his passions, or the impotent witnesses of his disorders, he imposes
them on him as a bridle, or opposes them to him as a dike:
Perfecti estote, "Be perfect," he tells us; a sublime saying,
which no legislator before him had pronounced, and none
since him has repeated. "Be perfect," not, like Aristides and
Cato, with that pagan perfection which, alongside the private
virtues which honor man, leaves intact all the vices which
oppress humanity;* but with the perfection of God himself,
that is to say, with that perfection which consists in obeying in
all things the most natural laws, which, being the enunciation
of the natural relationships of beings, are the expression of the
general will of their author; for that is the general or meta-
physical meaning of this passage: "Be perfect as your heavenly Father is perfect." And not only does he tell men, whom
he calls to the truth, to be better than the pagans: "For what
merit would you have," he asked them, "in doing what the
pagans do?", *None ethnici et hoc faciunt?,* but he tells them to
be better than the Jews themselves, the least imperfect of all
peoples; and he declares to them that "unless your justice
exceeds that of the scribes and Pharisees, you will surely not
enter the kingdom of heaven." He sets the difference between

---

*Cato was attending the abominable games of the goddess Flora; his pres-
ence disturbed the people. Cato noticed this, and departed to leave it every
license. Such was the virtue of the most virtuous of Roman magistrates.
Martial wrote an epigram on this event. These virtuous Romans attended
gladiatorial combats, sacrifices of human blood, when these took place;
suffered the exposure of children, etc., etc.

an imperfect and a perfect law before their eyes, when he tells them: "Your fathers were told to love those who loved them; but I tell you to love those who hate you." He presents the distinction between the *evil* works of the passions, the *imperfect* works of the law, and the *perfect* works of the love of one's neighbor, in the sublime parable where a man is *mistreated* by robbers, *neglected* by the Levite, and *rescued* by the Samaritan; for it is to be noted here that the Levite represents the imperfect state of the law, whose minister he is.

This mighty speech draws the social world from the nullity of error and the chaos of crime; order, or the unity of power, takes the place of the disorder of plurality in society. *Monotheism* in religion, *monogamy* in the family, and *monarchy* in the State little by little drive out *polytheism, polygamy,* and *polycracy,* or *popularism;* and, to remain with the subject at hand, marriage is recalled by the legislator himself to its institution of the *beginning,* that is to say, to its natural law; for nature is at the beginning of everything. Repudiation, even for the cause of adultery, is forbidden to men who did not even allege pretexts for divorce; and as far as voluptuous Egypt, where incest had been a political law and the means of royal succession, thousands of men renounced the most legitimate pleasures, in order to devote themselves with complete freedom to the contemplation of truth.

Mosaic law was thus accomplished in Christian law, and the perfection of laws and morals began for the universe. Judaic law, with its numerous practices, its minute observances, its wholly temporal punishments and rewards, was appropriate to society's childhood, that age in which a severe teacher rules all of man's steps, and speaks to him through his senses alone. Christian law, with its grand precepts, its universal morality, its eternal order of punishments and rewards, is appropriate to society's age of manhood, that age in which man, free inside the vast enclosure which society traces around him, contained in his passions by the laws, takes counsel for his duties from his heart alone. The one formed man for the domestic state of society, the society of self; the other formed him for the public state of society, the society of others. To prevent the Jew from harming his fellows, Moses forbade him to place a stumbling block in front of the blind man, required him to give directions to the stranger, and to help even the animal fallen under its burden. Jesus Christ goes further in a single word; he tells man, *Love your neighbor*. He makes this precept a commandment equal to the love for God himself, and he leaves it to the heart to direct the acts arising from it; and this is what made Saint Augustine say, *Ama, et fac quod vis;* "love, and do as you please."

I seem to see a child whose mother brings it into a group of people for the first time, and to which she gives beforehand all the little precepts of *childish civility,* under the hope of reward or threat of punishment proportional to its age; and a grown man whose sense of propriety alerts him to the politeness and consideration he owes others, in which he could not fail without covering himself with shame. Hence Moses formed a stubborn, fearful, and interested people, without vices, but above all without virtues; and Jesus Christ formed enlightened and strong nations, peoples, as the apostle says, acceptable to God and enamored of good works; *populum acceptabilem, sectatorem bonorum operum,*[1] in which morose minds see only the vices, because the virtues are the ordinary state and the only authorized one, as enthusiasts see only virtues in the pagans, because among them vice was the common state and allowed by the laws.

But the Christian religion in society, like truth and virtue in the heart of man, was a seed which time brought to maturity little by little. The convalescence of the world, if I dare say it, cured with so many pains of idolatry, was slow and laborious, and it long bore the scars of that great wound of humanity.

[1] Titus 2.14.

Infanticide, gladiatorial combats, blood-soaked sacrifices, and religious prostitution disappeared first from society; but slavery, superstition, divination, and above all divorce opposed a longer resistance to the influence of Christianity, and only gave way slowly before the progress of religious civilization. The Eastern emperors, with their precarious and contested authority, did not dare to deliver society from it, and limited themselves to restraining or regulating its practice. The Frankish kings, up to the third dynasty, still practiced repudiation, which is found in the infancy of all societies. They were corrected in this by the common father of Christians, who taught the peoples by recalling half-barbarian kings to the severity of Christianity, and making these proud Sicambrians bow their heads; and even in our time, the dispensations for certain degrees of kinship in marriage, sometimes lightly accorded (for which cause the proposed Civil Code abolishes this law), were a remnant of condescension for human weakness, which the advanced state of society should perhaps have caused to disappear, especially in France, where the law excluding women from the succession to the throne meant that dispensations of this kind were never politically necessary. I do not fear to guarantee that law in France will become severe in proportion as license has been excessive, and that this maxim of M. de Montesquieu: "In France, troubles have always strengthened power," will sooner or later, in the Church as in the State, receive the widest application. And has Europe not already seen ecclesiastical discipline reestablished in the Christian world by the Council of Trent, following the license introduced by the Reformation, and, in all States, the police laws becoming more severe in the aftermath of civil troubles? For order, in society under the name of civilization, in man under the name of reason, is the natural state of beings: "order," says Fr. Malebranche, "is the inviolable law of minds."

CHAPTER 9

Revolution in Christian Society

FOR over ten centuries, marriage in Europe had been constituted on the natural law of indissolubility. Paternity or power
was *honored* in the family as in the State, as in religion. Society
was advancing, with the help of Christianity, in the knowledge
of truth and the practice of good. "France," says M. de Saint-
Lambert, who cannot be suspected of partiality in favor of
Christianity, "was in that period the country where justice was
best administered, and in which the magistrates had the
minds, characters, and morals which they should have had.
Their power offended none; it contributed to the security of
all. . . . The nation was acquiring all those habits which, in a
society, become virtues or the support of virtues. At these
times, the morals of the French may have been comparable to
the finest morals of the illustrious nations of antiquity.* . . .
Religion was conducive to order and morals; the religious
troubles which arose forced the government to suspend the
execution of its useful designs, and to oppose the new opinions."

Such was the state of society in France, and in many regards
in Christian Europe, when the great scandal of the Reformation came to halt, or rather suspend, the natural development
of society in the perfecting of its laws, and to return religion to
the imperfect state, to the hard, interested, and fearful spirit of
the Judaic religion, and domestic and political society to the

---

*One senses that a philosopher who sees the perfection of morals among the
Greeks and Romans, where he sees the perfection of the arts, could offer no
higher compliment.

vicious institutions of the Greeks, whose arts, carried to Europe in this period, made no small contribution to the admiration and adoption of their laws.

"Luther," says the author cited above, "was not a man of genius, yet he changed the world"; which is to say that he altered man and overturned society. By a remarkable contradiction, the Reformation introduced laxity into society's principles and rigidity into man's morals; for those same doctors who allowed the dissolution of the conjugal tie condemned with a fierce austerity the most innocent recreation on Sunday, which for them was the *Sabbath* day; and the religious troubles of England and Scotland offer laughable examples of this.

Thus while Luther, and still more Calvin, taught the despairing or corrupting dogmas of absolute predestination to eternal damnation, or those of inamissible justice, and while denying at once human weakness and divine grace, they distinguished men into two classes, one of the just who cannot err, another of the wicked who cannot improve themselves, they brought confusion into society, by setting plurality or democracy in the place of unity everywhere: democracy in the family, by the faculty of divorce accorded to women; democracy in the State, by the sovereign power attributed to the people; democracy in religion, by the authority conveyed to the faithful for the election of ministers, and even in every man, for the interpretation of the Scriptures: "For," M. de Saint-Lambert naively says, "Calvin's Christian is necessarily a democrat." And then began, for Europe, the revolution from natural or divine laws to vicious and unnatural ones, a work of man and his passions; a revolution which at the time of its origin incited such bloody wars, which engendered such monstrous errors and such unbelievable crimes; which, combined with the progress of commerce and the arts, that is to say, with the thirst for gain and the lust for pleasure, has raised the same tempests in man's heart it has excited in society, and produced disgust in living for virtue in those who can no longer live for the pleasures: for suicide, which has become so common in our midst, and will soon leave no more criminals for human justice to punish, only dates in Europe from the times of which I speak; and it is the same doctrines which have given man the power to destroy himself, and which have taught, by the voice of the philosopher of Geneva, that "the people always has the right to change its laws, even the best ones; for if it wishes to harm itself, who has the right to prevent it from doing so?"

But the mightiest vehicle of license and disorder was the faculty of divorce, which Luther thought he had found in the gospel; for in this epoch of society, the reason for political laws was still sought in religion. The lights of good sense alone should have taught him that he who had *come to accomplish the law* of the Jews, and to say to men: "Be perfect as your heavenly Father is perfect," had not meant to leave them under the imperfect law of the Jews, let alone a much more imperfect law than that of the Jews; since, as we have already observed, repudiation is a harsh law, and mutual divorce a bad law; and since, in the same sermon* in which, opposing the imperfect elements of a law given to children to the perfection of the same law developed and accomplished for grown men, Jesus Christ says to the Jews: "You have been told: You shall not kill, and I tell you not even to utter an angry word against your brother. You have been told: You shall not commit adultery, and I tell you not even to look upon a woman lustfully. You have been told not to hate your enemies, and I tell you to love your enemies, and to do good to those who hate you"; in this same sermon, I say, it is supremely absurd to suppose that this teacher of all perfection meant to say to the Jews: "Moses allowed husbands to repudiate their wives, and I allow wives to repudiate their husbands." He should have learned from this gospel, which gives him the lie as many times as he invokes it, that Jesus Christ, questioned by the Jews on the

*Saint Matth. ch. 5.

meaning of the law of Moses relative to the dissolution of the conjugal tie, could only speak to them of the kind of dissolution tolerated by Moses, that is to say, of repudiation exercised by the husband alone; and indeed, the divine legislator uses only the expressions *dimittere uxorem, uxorem dimissam*[1] to express the dissolution of the conjugal tie, and the wife separated from her husband; and that Saint Paul, who is speaking only to Christians, and who undoubtedly understood the meaning of the gospel, says: "If a woman marries another man during the life of her husband, she will be held an adulteress; but if her husband dies, she is freed of this law, and can marry another without adultery"; and that finally, if this passage in the gospel is addressed to Christians, it signifies only separation *a mensa et a toro,* for the cause of adultery: a separation which honor commands and reason allows. For the rest, I shall not discuss this passage in the gospel, since those whom I am combating do not oppose it to us; and since, in addition, they have gone far beyond the bounds which, according to Luther and Calvin, the legislator of the Christians assigned to the faculty of dissolving the matrimonial tie.

In any event, mutual divorce had only been practiced for a few years when we see *Stör, Müntzer, Karlstadt,* some of Luther's first and most zealous disciples, reproaching him for having introduced a *dissolution similar to that of Mohammedanism;* and indeed, divorce had even then begun to transform itself into polygamy. Luther himself constantly had these famous words on his lips: *Si nolit uxor, ancilla venito.*[2] This patriarch of the Reformation, assisted by his learned doctors, allowed the Landgrave of Hesse, by his consultation of December, 1539, to marry a second wife, while retaining his first one; and similarly, in our own time, the late king of Prussia, Frederick William II, repudiated Elizabeth of Brunswick, mar-

[1] "To send a wife away," "a wife who has been sent away."
[2] "If the wife is unwilling, let the maid come in."

ried the princess of Hesse, married the countess of Enhoff, without repudiating the queen, in each case with the approval of the Calvinist doctors; and when, with these three women still living, he wished to marry Mademoiselle de Voss, he found his pastors disposed to grant their permission, alleging that it was better to contract an illegitimate marriage than to run endlessly from error to error; a derisory and shameful decision, which "degrades those who render it as much as he who requests it," says with reason M. de Ségur, recent historian of this memorable moment of our time.

CHAPTER 10

Of the French Revolution

BEFORE the present revolution, divorce in France, allowed to some by their religious law, was forbidden to all by the civil law; but the civil law allowed spouses separation, examples of which, unheard of formerly, became more common in proportion as morals became weaker. This condescension of the legislator, or rather of the magistrates, who were not restrained by certain conditions necessary to prevent its abuse, had borne bitter fruit for fifty years; and legal separations, or merely *de facto* ones, lightly pronounced by the courts, or indiscreetly tolerated by the police, had disposed men's minds to accept the faculty of divorce as a necessary remedy, while at the same time other principles, widespread in all classes of society, had prepared the citizens to receive popular institutions without horror, and as philosophical conceptions. But divorce and democracy, introduced after such a long experience of natural constitution of family and State, in what was, through the habit of several centuries of reason and nature, the most enlightened and indeed the strongest society in Europe, presumed a prodigious obscuring of enlightenment, an extreme weakness in souls, and were bound to produce far more unhappy effects than they had at a more distant time among far less constituted peoples. That is what happened; and without speaking here of the public disorders in laws and morals at a certain time in our revolution, which exceed anything imaginable, the number of divorces in the first three months of 1793, though only in Paris, was equal to one-third the number of marriages. Divorce is perhaps less frequent today in one locale, but it is more widespread, and already it is reaching the countryside. At first it was an object of horror there, soon it will no longer even be a subject of attention. One must not forget to observe that most divorces are provoked by women; which proves that they are weaker or more impassioned, not that they are more unhappy.

It is above all in the revolution effected in France that there have appeared, with all their characteristics, the intimate union and perfect analogy between the two societies, domestic and public. Thus the Constituent Assembly established popular sovereignty as a principle in the State, and even in the Church, by the democratico-royal Constitution of 1789 and the Civil or Presbyterian Constitution of the Clergy; and by doing so it opened the road to divorce, which allows the wife to usurp power over her husband; so that the Legislative Assembly which followed, in decreeing divorce, had merely to deduce a consequence. Scarcely had natural relationships been inverted than the degeneration increased with horrifying speed. The year 1793 witnessed, in the State, the most unrestrained demagogy; in the family, the most unlimited dissolution of the conjugal tie; in religion itself, the most execrable impiety. Paternal power perished along with marital authority; the minority of children was shortened, and by the forced equality of shares in inheritance, the father lost the safeguard of authority, the means to punish and reward.

Nevertheless the excess of disorder brings a return to the rule, and the edifice is rebuilt with its own ruins. It was sought, to avail myself of Montesquieu's expression in speaking of Rome, *to remove the republic from the hands of the people,* and at the same time to remove the family from the hands of women and children. The Directorial Constitution restricted the overly broad democracy; some limits were imposed on the license of divorce; the father obtained permission to dipose of some portion of his goods; and the Directory even returned, under onerous conditions, a shadow of tolerance to religious worship.

The 18th Brumaire arrived;[1] and the political constitution which resulted from the events of that memorable day brings a principle of unity into the State, gives more freedom to the ministers of religious worship, and even the Civil Code, which is the object of this discussion, seeks to reconstitute domestic power, rendering marital power better defended against divorce, and paternal power freer in the disposition of domestic property.

I shall not dwell further on the sequels to the events of the 18th Brumaire; but the reader is now in a position to evaluate these two assertions by the author of the *Spirit of the Laws:* first, that divorce ordinarily has great political utility; second, that society's public state has no relationship to its domestic state.

We shall conclude with some general considerations on divorce.

---

[1] Napoleon Bonaparte's coup d'état (November 9, 1799).

CHAPTER 11

General Considerations on Divorce

THE repudiation tolerated among the Jews was a harsh law, wholly to the advantage of the husband against the wife, which made the former a despot and the latter a slave. It is consequently unsuited to Christian peoples, whose first law is charity, and among which marriage, returned to the institution of the *beginning,* makes woman, not a being equal to man, but a *helper* (or minister) *similar to him.*

Divorce is both a harsh and a false law, because it not only allows the husband the faculty of repudiating his wife, but also grants it to the wife against her husband.

Today more than ever, divorce is a weak or oppressive law for both sexes, because it delivers them to the depravity of their penchants, at the very time that the passions, exalted by the progress of the arts, most need to be contained by the severity of the laws.

Divorce is only tolerated among commercial peoples because they picture domestic society, and even political society, as a commercial association, a social contract. This is only a play on words, an illusion which vanishes under the slightest scrutiny.

Domestic society is not a commercial association, which the partners enter with equal stakes and can leave with equal results. It is a society to which the man brings the protection of strength, the woman, the needs of weakness; one power, the other duty; a society which the man enters with authority, the woman with dignity; which the man leaves with all his authority, but the woman cannot leave with all her dignity: for out of everything she brought into the society, she can only, in the event of dissolution, recover her money. And is it not supremely unjust that the woman, having entered the family with youth and fertility, may leave it with sterility and old age, and that, belonging only to the domestic state, she should be put out of the family to which she gave existence, at the time in life when nature denies her the ability to begin another one?

Marriage is therefore not an ordinary contract, since in terminating it, the two parties cannot return themselves to the same state they were in before entering into it. And if the contract is voluntary at the time it is entered into, it can no longer be voluntary, and almost never is, at the time of its termination, since the party which manifests the desire to dissolve it takes all liberty from the other party to refuse, and has only too many means to force its consent.

And admire here the inconsistency into which the proposed Civil Code falls. It is not a question, it says, of knowing whether the faculty of divorce is good in itself, but of "whether it is appropriate that the laws should induce the coactive power to intervene in a matter which is naturally so free, and in which the heart must play so great a role." And elsewhere: "marital society is unlike any other; mutual consent cannot dissolve marriage,* even though it may dissolve every other society." Thus the law itself recognizes so little freedom in this *matter which is naturally so free,* and so little power in the parties to dissolve, even by their consent, a union formed by their consent, that the proof of their mutual agreement to dissolve the union is a cause which prevents its dissolution, and their collusion in this regard is an offense punishable by a fine; so that in order to form the association, it was necessary to prove the mutual consent of the two parties, while in order to break it, it is necessary to prove that the two parties do not consent to the rupture; as if their agreement in wishing to

*The Civil Code allows the dissolution of marriage by mutual consent of the spouses.

separate were not the strongest proof the law could desire of the absence of all affection, and the need for a separation.

Divorce, which may in some cases favor the perpetuity of a family, is contrary to the conservation of the human species; because spouses who wish to divorce will have no children, in order to acquire a ground for divorce, and because the neglect in which divorce too often leaves children impairs their conservation, even when a second marriage does not endanger their lives; and as a society is made up of those who subsist, and not those who are born, if polygamy causes more children to be born, monogamy conserves more of them.

But if nature does not wish the bond of marriage ever to be dissolved, does not society demand that it may be dissolved on occasion?

A society in its first youth has no other passion than war. It is a growing child, whose chief desire is for the exercise necessary to its physical development. At this age, the conjugal tie's dissolubility is without danger, because its dissolution is without example; and indeed on occasion, as among the Jews, dissolubility is tolerated in order to encourage the multiplication of a nascent people.

But the age of puberty comes for society as for man, and the passions acquire a different character. In the first age, man made war on man; in the second, he makes war on woman; and voluptuousness oppresses one sex as war had destroyed the other. The advances of civilization awaken the taste for pleasure, and the arts dispute the care of its embellishment: everything becomes art, even nature; and the very needs of humanity are no longer anything but artificial pleasures, which man pursues ardently, and often at the expense of his fellows. At this age of society, to allow the dissolution of the conjugal tie is to require its dissolution. The law cannot authorize divorce then without introducing a limitless polygamy for both sexes. A nation which has public pleasures, and even public women, requires a public bridle as well and public laws, en-

tirely general, entirely imperative, which maintain general
order among all, and not laws which in a sense are private,
which legislate only for a particular order of circumstances;
laws of dispensation, expedient for the passions and weaknesses of a few.

Thus, to whatever side man leans, the law must right him;
and today it must forbid dissolution to dissolute men, as a few
centuries ago it forbade private vengeance to fierce and vindic-
tive men; and it is only in this improvement of the laws, and
not in the progress of the arts, that consists the perfectibility of
the human species, over which men only argue because they
fail to understand each other.

Moreover, if there were legitimate grounds for divorce, they
would be those which arise from nature itself, like those bodily
infirmities which lie outside the realm of human will, and
which man has no means to prevent; and it is for this reason
that the law of the Jews made them grounds for repudiation.
But to allow spouses to leave each other when, delivered by
the very hope of divorce to the inconstancy of their tastes and
the violence of their penchants, they have established adulterous loves elsewhere; to dissolve their union, because they do
not wish to control their humors, or the law does not wish to
watch over their conduct; to allow them to break the bond,
when they have loosened it by a voluntary absence, is to
weaken will, deprave actions, disorder man (and laws are no
more required to disorder than plans to destroy); it is to place
the family and State in a false and unnatural position, because
the family must then oppose the strength of its morals to the
weakness of the law, instead of finding in the law a support
against the weakness of its morals. But where the law is weak,
the rule of morals is falsified, and there is no more remedy for
their inevitable corruption; and where the law is strong, public
authority has a fixed, immutable rule, by which it can always
maintain morals or rectify them.

If the dissolution of the conjugal tie is allowed, even for the cause of adultery, all women who wish to divorce will render themselves guilty of adultery; women will be a commodity in circulation; and the accusation of adultery will be the common currency, and the accepted medium for all exchanges; for this is the point of corruption which man has reached in England; and in the debates which took place not long ago in Parliament on the need to restrain the faculty of divorce, the Bishop of Rochester, replying to Lord Mulgrave, claimed that out of ten requests for divorce on the ground of adultery—for one divorces in England on this basis alone—there were nine in which the seducer had agreed in advance with the husband to provide him with evidence of his wife's infidelity.*

This is the place to observe that, in a case of adultery between persons of the highest rank which was recently argued in England,† Lord Kenyon, the oracle of the law, who presided at the trial, in the summation of the case which he presented to the judges, attenuated the offenses of the wife and even those of her seducer in consideration of similar offenses on the part of the husband; and as a form of compensation, reduced the damages requested by the latter against the seducer to a hundred pounds sterling.

Nothing better demonstrates than such a decision to what an extent the social ideas of justice, and even of honor, are perverted in this mercantile nation. In effect, it presumes

---

*The same orator maintains that the men in England who were the most indulgent toward divorce were also the most extreme partisans of French demagogy. The Civil Code forbids a woman divorced on the ground of adultery to remarry her accomplice. This restriction jeopardizes the life of the husband: there is nothing more dangerous than to compromise thusly with the passions, to allow them to go to a certain point in order to halt them afterward.

†Mr. Sturt, a member of the English Parliament, against the marquess of Blanford, eldest son of the Duke of Marlborough, for adultery committed with Anne Sturt, daughter of the earl of Shaftesbury. At the same time, another suit brought by the honorable Mr. Windham, His Brittanic Majesty's minister to Florence, against Earl Wycombe, eldest son of the marquess of Lansdowne.

natural equality of offenses, and hence of duties, between husband and wife; but the infidelity of the wife dissolves the domestic tie, because it introduces foreign children into the family; whereas the disorders of the husband, however great they may be, have no consequences for the family, and can afflict only the heart of the wife.*

The decision of which I speak demonstrates the extreme degradation of morals in England, where a husband, even in the highest ranks and the most opulent circumstances, does not blush to receive the price of his dishonor, and can speculate in advance on the infidelity of his wife, and come to terms with the fortune of her seducer.† It is by the same principle that in cases of intent to duel, the law in England requires the two parties to post a pecuniary bond that they will not come to fight, and there is a recent example of this. There were, in France, more correct ideas, and above all more upright morals: the individual notified of an intent to duel posted a bond of honor for his deference to the law; and an outraged spouse, even in the last classes of the people, would have been marked with infamy if he had sought a pecuniary reparation in the courts.

---

*"We see," says the abbé de Rastignac, "in a canon of the second letter of Saint Basil to Amphilocus, that the customary canonical penalties were less severe toward men than toward women, in the very case where men and women were guilty of the same sin."

†The situation is roughly the same among a number of savage peoples, where the husband requires a lover found with his wife to pay a roast pig, and eats it with them. The principle is the same, the currency used is of no importance. One finds in the English, under the brilliant exterior of refinement and progress in the arts, many of the characteristics of savage peoples: the practice of theft, the passion for strong liquors, the taste for half-cooked meat without bread, the imperfection of the laws, etc., etc. "A son, barely out of adolescence," says the *Essay on Paternal Power,* "was called to testify against his father; his deposition completed the evidence of a capital crime, and his father's death sentence practically came from his mouth. This decision was handed down at the latest assizes at Carrikfergus; the accused was named William Mowens."

Commerce in society is what the natural need to eat and drink is in man. Man cannot make eating and drinking his principal concern without falling into the deepest degradation and totally forgetting his duties. A people which places commerce in the rank of social institutions, which sees a duty in it rather than a need, which, by every means possible, gives it an unlimited extension, instead of enclosing it within the bounds of the indispensably necessary, may dazzle by the brilliance of its enterprises and the magnitude of its successes; but its physical prosperity conceals degraded souls and abject morals: it is a wholly material people, and will sooner or later be subjugated by a moral people. In France, the frenzy for commerce was contained by institutions which forbade its practice to certain classes of society,* and which maintained the spirit of detachment from riches, and the disposition to leave everything in order to fulfill one's duties. In this lay the strength of France; and if the Revolution had permanently destroyed its principle, the French would have been sufficiently punished, and their enemies sufficiently revenged.

Just as adultery is the sole means of divorce in England, so incompatibility of temperament, which is decreed as a ground for divorce by existing law, and is once again being requested by the Court of Cassation, would be the common means for those who had no other in France; and already one sees this incompatibility alleged by all spouses who wish to separate, even those in whom the public can reproach nothing except the excessive compatibility of their tastes, and a vile complaisance in their mutual disorders.

It must be observed that the authors of the Civil Code, who set themselves, and rightly so, against the ground of *incompatibility of temperament,* which currently suffices to effect

*That is why certain persons in France could not, without dishonoring themselves, sign agreements which might subject them to physical constraint, because their persons, already committed to the service of society, could not be alienated to the individual.

the dissolution of the conjugal tie, allow that dissolution *when the habitual conduct of one spouse toward the other makes life unbearable for the latter;* a ground which strongly resembles that of incompatibility, and which spouses can always allege, because no one can contradict them.

And note here the impropriety, to say no more, of a law which allows the formation of new bonds by a woman convicted of having violated her first commitment by adultery, and which thereby rewards the neglect of duty and the infraction of the law; for in a well-regulated State, marriage, allowed to all men, should be forbidden to divorced spouses, for the same reason that careers in public administration, accessible to all citizens, are irrevocably closed to those who have been negligent or dishonest in the exercise of their functions.

Thus, in the earliest times, the interdiction of marriage was one of the canonical penalties inflicted by the Church on those guilty of murder or incest; and this penalty could still be successfully employed by a vigilant administration. Even if one considers celibacy a penalty, a spouse who has distanced a guilty woman from himself, and is prevented from marrying another, would not always be unjustly punished, because the faults of the wife are too often those of the husband, and almost always indict his interested or frivolous choice, his tyrannical humor, his weak conduct, or his bad example.

The proposed Civil Code, to be sure, takes away with one hand what it gives with the other. At the same time that it allows the faculty of divorce, it hinders its exercise; but it is here above all that the law appears defective, and the remedy inadequate and derisory.

The legislator declares marriage dissoluble: there ends his action; it is up to domestic persons to apply the law to each other. Only they can be the judges of domestic offenses, because only they can have cognizance of them, and because the intimate conviction which is born for each of them, even from his suspicions and fears, is equivalent, for a domestic offense, to the conviction which the magistrate charged with the pursuit of public offenses must seek from external witnesses.

Indeed, of the five causes which the proposed Civil Code specifies for divorce, only two, *public defamation* and *the desertion of one party by the other*, can be subject to a public proof, because both of these offenses occur outside the domestic enclosure; and this is so true that defamation in front of servants only, or desertion between two spouses who remain in the same household, separated and with no communication between them, which is possible and even frequent, would not be admitted as grounds for a request of divorce, even if the two parties lived at the opposite ends of a park several miles long, as long as they were within the same enclosure; because in this case, neither the defamation nor the desertion, though real, would be public. But as for the other three causes, the most common and most serious of all: (1) habitual conduct which makes life in common unbearable; (2) the attempted murder of one spouse by the other; (3) adultery; "Where," rightly demands, in its opinion, the Court of Cassation—which, consistent with its principles, wishes that if the law allows divorce, the will of one party should suffice to obtain it—"Where is a fact which a husband or wife can present in evidence? Where is one which they can prove? Where is one which can be judged?" A woman will have victoriously proved her innocence before the courts, only to be irrevocably condemned by her husband, and often by the public as well; the judges will have seen no proof of the husband's foul temper, while his wife is convinced it is unbearable. They will sometimes see only sweetness and submission where there is an intent and attempt to murder; *the sacred character of virtue will shine for them on the brow of a profane adulterer.* And certainly no tyranny is less reasonable and at the same time more ridiculous than that of a magistrate who, interposing himself between a husband and wife discontented with each other, comes to investigate their mutual affections, in order coldly to judge the degree of their reciprocal alienation; who advises hate it should love, counsels frenzy to calm itself, prescribes delays to impatience, and deliberateness to passion, denies jealousy its suspicions,* and the heart itself its wound, and appears to tell spouses who are reciprocally accusing each other of murder and adultery: "Wait; you are not yet divided enough for me to separate you."

The faculty of divorce is to be hindered by the long and expensive forms of procedure which accompany its request and delay its pronouncement. But has sufficient consideration been given to the drawbacks of an enabling law which, because of the difficulty of its execution, will be enabling for the passions and weaknesses of the rich only, that is, of those who generally have less violent passions and more compatible temperaments, because education and etiquette have taught them to restrain these? Will the faculty of divorce be like those spectacles where the rich enter for a high price, and seat themselves conveniently, while the poor man, who also wants to see, besieges the roofs and windows; and is it not evident that where some divorce on the strength of money, others will divorce on the strength of crimes?

In the course of this work, I have often compared divorce as practiced among the Christians to polygamy as practiced in the Orient, because divorce is in fact a form of genuine polygamy. The Protestant authors themselves do not consider it otherwise; and Theodore Beza begins thus his *Treatise of Polygamy and Divorce,* published in Deventer:

> I call polygamy the plurality of marriages; and there are two kinds of it: either the same man is married to several women at once, or, the preceding marriage having been dissolved, he marries a different woman.†

---

*Molière has placed this subject on the stage twice, in *Georges Dandin* and in *Tartuffe,* where Mme. Pernelle insists on denying what Orgon so pleasantly assures her he has *seen.*

†*Polygamiam voco conjugii multiplicationem, cujus duae sunt species. Vel enim uno eodemque tempore plures uxores ducuntur, aut soluto matrimonio alia uxor ducitur.* Tractatio de Polygamia et Divortiis. Deventer.[1]

[1] Theodore Beza, *Tractatio de Polygamia et Divortiis* (Daventriae: typis J. Columbii, 1651; orig. ed. 1568).

In the early days of the Reformation, the courts considered divorce to be a tacit toleration of polygamy. One finds in a collection of decisions[2] the following case, cited in condensed form in Le Brun's *Journal of Jurisprudence*:[3]

T. Gautier and Jacquette Pourceau, husband and wife, after a *de facto* separation, each remarried a different person. The governor of La Rochelle condemned them to be exposed for two hours in front of the palace, each attached to a collar, the man with two distaffs, the woman with two hats. They were enjoined to resume living together, and forbidden to live with or remarry others, on pain of death. This sentence was confirmed by a decree given at the Chamber of Edicts on November 23, 1606.

And this sentence, adds the commentator, *was so moderate, given that the accused were of the pretended reformed religion.* M. Le Brun's *Journal* reports this case, or a similar one, as follows: "According to an ancient commentator," he says, "N. and his wife, convicted of bigamy at the Parlement of Paris, were only condemned to exposition, given that they were Calvinists, and their law allows divorce"; which means that bigamy and polygamy, which our laws punished by a capital sentence, appeared to the courts more worthy of excuse among men whose religion allowed them the dissolution of the conjugal tie. Thus the police would not tolerate the public practice of polygamy by Orientals living in France; but the laws would not punish them for having practiced it, and would see in it only a consequence of their morals and laws.

But if the polygamy of the Orientals is as unhappy in its consequences for the family as divorce, divorce is in general more dangerous to the State. In effect, polygamy leaves children with those who have given them life, while divorce forcibly separates them from one or the other of them. Polygamy enclosed within the privacy of the family is practiced without

[2] Probably Pierre Le Brun, *Recueil de causes célèbres,* 24 vols. (Paris: 1801–1803).

[3] *Journal de jurisprudence* (Paris: Académie de législation, pub. 1801–1806).

disturbance or scandal; divorce makes the courts resound with its complaints, and entertains the idleness of circles with its indiscreet revelations. The Turks buy their neighbor's daughter; we, with divorce, carry off our friend's wife. In the Orient, women are reserved: "Nothing equals," says M. de Montesquieu, "the modesty of Turkish and Persian women." Wherever the faculty of divorce allows a woman to see a possible husband in every man, the women are without shame, or at least without delicacy, because the plurality of men, which is the sequel to divorce, is more contrary to nature and public morals than the plurality of women allowed to men by the polygamy of the Orient. "If one leaves," says Mme. Necker, "married women the freedom to make a new choice, soon their glances will wander over all men, and soon only the privilege of perjury will distinguish them from actresses, who have a right to preferences and a taste for changes."

Beside all these natural reasons in favor of the indissolubility of the conjugal tie, what are all the human motives which can be alleged to justify the faculty of dissolving it? What does it matter, after all, if a few individuals suffer in the course of this transient life, as long as reason, nature, and society do not suffer? And if man sometimes bears with regret a chain he cannot break, does he not suffer at all moments of his life, from his passions which he cannot subdue, from his inconstancy which he cannot settle; and is the entire life of man anything but a continual struggle against his penchants? It is up to man to harmonize tempers and characters in marriage, and to forestall disorders in the family by the equanimity of his temper and the wisdom of his conduct. But when he has made his choice against all the laws of reason, and solely on the basis of whim or interest, when he has founded his life's happiness on what only makes for the pleasure of a few moments, when he himself has poisoned the sweetness of a reasonable union by weak or unjust conduct; unhappy through his own fault, has he the right to ask society to take responsibility for his errors and offenses? Must one dissolve the family in order to contrive new pleasures for his passions, or new opportunities for his inconstancy, and corrupt an entire people because of the corruption of a few?

How much wiser is the Christian religion! It forbids men the love of riches and pleasures, prolific cause of ill-assorted marriages; it orders children to follow the advice of their parents in this, the most important act of their lives. Once the union is established, it commands support to the strongest, gentleness to the weakest, virtue to all. It continually interposes itself to avert discontents and end disputes. But if, in spite of its exhortations, faults and vices transform the lifelong bond into a daily misery, then it loosens it, but without breaking it. It separates the bodies, but without dissolving the society; and leaving embittered humors the time to soften themselves, it encourages hearts in the hope and ease of reunion; and this religion, which forbids everything to the passions, and pardons everything to fragility; this religion, which commands the guilty man to hope in the benevolence of his creator, does not wish the rash or frivolous woman to despair of her husband's affection. Philosophy raises divorce between the spouses like an impenetrable wall; religion places separation between them like an officious veil. Philosophy, which rejects all means of grace and remission from human society* as from religion, irrevocably stigmatizes a woman more weak than guilty, by the indelible mark of divorce which it prints on her brow; and taking from her the dignity of a wife, which a second union cannot return to her, and with which, as Tacitus says, one compromises once and for life, *cum spe votoque uxoris semel transigitur*,[4] it delivers her defenseless to all the inconstancy of her penchants; but the doctrine of he who pardoned the

*The philosophers who governed or inspired the revolution in France, in giving the people the right to condemn, took from the king the right to pardon.
[4] "Once married, they no longer hope and pray [for another marriage]." Tacitus, *Germany* 19.2.

adulteress, more indulgent to human weakness, conserves her husband's name to the unfaithful party, at the very moment that, through separation, men take away her rights as a wife, and still keeps watch over the honor of she who did not take care of her happiness.

It is up to the civil law to do the rest; and separations, which have been so common for some time, would be much less frequent if the law imposed conditions on the separated spouses which made them a penalty for all, and an indulgence for none.

And, for example, any woman separated from her husband, even for violence and ill-treatment, should in the future retire into the bosom of a religious society, the only society to which she still belongs. This refuge, open to repentance, to weakness, to unhappiness, would afford her, in a more intimate union with Divinity, the only consolations which a virtuous woman forsaken by an unjust husband should seek and may enjoy; or would cause to disappear from society the scandal of a being outside its natural place, of a wife who is no longer in the dependence of her husband, and of a mother who exercises no further authority over her children, and whose conduct, too often equivocal, like her existence, carries into others' families the trouble she has brought into her own. It would be equally necessary, and extremely useful to public morals, that every man separated from his wife be obliged to renounce and prohibited from aspiring to any public function, because it is indispensable for the family that the head exercise authority in it himself when he no longer has a *minister* to exercise it for him; and, above all, because it is important to teach men that public functions do not dispense them from domestic virtues. This law, a very natural one, would be more effective against the abuse of separations than against the faculty of divorce.

Perhaps the law should also consider separated spouses as deceased parents, in which case it would appoint a guardian for their children, if they have property, or, if they have none, it would entrust their education to the administration which, gathering them into the public establishments, would remove them from the misery of seeing themselves torn between disunited parents, to be raised in the hatred of a father or the contempt of a mother, heirs to their mutual resentments, and condemned to perpetuate them in fraternal hatreds.

It is necessary to reply to certain objections. The partisans of divorce put forth the example of Poland, where the Catholic religion allows divorce, and that of the Protestant countries, which practice divorce, it is said, without inconvenience; and it is even claimed that morals are better there than in countries where divorce is forbidden.

1. It is a waste of argument to claim that the dissolution of the conjugal tie, formed with all the conditions required for its validity, is allowed in Poland; and in order not to interrupt the train of these reflections with overly long citations, the documents are placed at the end of the work which formally establish the falsity of this opinion, which informed men can no longer allow themselves to maintain.*

These documents make it clear that marriage is indissoluble in Poland, as in other Catholic States, but that the grounds for annulment there are more common or more lightly pronounced; and this is a last proof, but in my view a conclusive and decisive one, of the principle so often repeated in this work of the homogeneity of the two societies, domestic and public, religious and physical, and of the analogy of their respective constitutions in every nation. In effect, as Poland is the only monarchical State in Europe which has been unable to attain its natural constitution, even the Catholic family is less strongly constituted there than in other States of the same religion, and Christianity itself is divided among a mixture of Greeks, Jews, Socinians, Anabaptists, and even occult sects which are suspected of having arisen in that unhappy country

*See the Appendix at the end of the work.

and of continuing to make their homes there. Unfortunate nation, which, having some centuries ago fallen back into the state of childhood, has perished in wishing to return to manhood!

2. Morals, it is said, are better in Protestant countries than in Catholic States. This assertion, repeated a thousand times by the many enemies of Christianity, requires some development; and it is here that one must distinguish the weakness of man from the weakness of the laws.

License in man's morals, it is true, was born in Italy, from the progress of the arts, necessary sequel to the progress of commerce, encouraged by princes whom it had enriched and enthroned; but license in the very rules of morality, or in the laws, began in the North, with the opinions of Luther, supported by princes avid for novelties and riches. The disorders in Italy were personal and sought the shadow of mystery; in Germany they were public and authorized; and while the Italian plotted an intrigue to seduce his neighbor's wife, the German carried her off by the decision of a judge, and married her in the presence of a notary; and this is what the Germans call the *blessed Reformation,* as we spoke in '90 of *our superb Constitution.* Soon, if Luther's most zealous disciples must be believed, the dissolution of morals, infallible sequel to such laws, reached the highest pitch in Germany, and was *comparable to the license of Mohammedanism;* and we have already seen that Luther himself allowed polygamy to the Landgrave of Hesse, but in great secrecy, and indeed under the seal of confession, *sub sigillo confessionis.**

---

*The extremely curious consultation of the Landgrave of Hesse, and the no less curious decision of Luther and seven other famous doctors of his party, were published in 1679 by the Prince Palatine, in authentic form, along with the document of the second marriage. They are found in the *History of the Variations.*[5]

[5] Jacques-Bénigne Bossuet (bishop of Meaux), *Histoire des variations des églises protestantes* (Paris: la veuve de S. Mabre-Cramoisy, 1688; various subsequent editions).

The Christian religion was thus being attacked at the two extremes of the Christian world at the same time, in man's morals and society's laws, when the Christian world was attacked in its territory by the arms of the Ottoman empire, which were so formidable at the time. These two causes of disorder, license in the arts and weakness in the laws, have since marched in tandem in society, until the moment when modern philosophy, which is made up at once of the weakest opinions on laws and the most decided taste for the arts, had combined in France, as in a hearth placed in the center of Europe, these two principles of domestic and public disorder; a horrid combination, whose violent explosion has reacted against both the North and South; like those terrible detonations produced suddenly by the mixture of two liquors.

The arts of the South had penetrated to the North, although slowly, in the wake of the riches produced by commerce; but in the South, political and religious causes had prevented the propagation of the principles of the Reformation. There was thus an additional principle of license in Protestant than in Catholic Europe; and how could reason admit that more numerous causes should produce fewer effects, especially if one considers that the Catholic religion, with its *sensible* cult and irksome practices, imposes a more present and severe restraint on our passions, at the same time that it offers us, in the austere rules of certain institutions, always stronger than men, models of detachment from all the pleasures?

I therefore do not fear to affirm that there have long been more disorders of the kind in question among Protestant peoples than in Catholic States: I say the peoples; for where, as in France, there are only individuals mingled with a numerous Catholic population, no difference in habits is visible. I shall cite in support of my assertion Major *Weiss,* a senator of Bern, known for his attachment to the French Revolution, whose progress he sought, too late, to prevent in his homeland, and who displays an extreme bias in favor of the Protestant nations in his writings. "The two most *manly* nations in Europe," he says in his *Philosophical Principles*,[6] "the English and the Prussian, are those where the weaknesses of love are treated with the most indulgence."* Among the English, the theater is of a revolting indecency, and M. Hugh Blair, celebrated professor of literature at Edinburgh, notes that the French in particular are shocked by it. Berlin is the most corrupt city in Europe. In Geneva, license in principles had long ago triumphed over rigorism in forms, and there were more disorders than in any other city in France of the same rank. Morals in France were good in the countryside, and at least decent in the cities. There are departments where, even today, divorce is unheard of and the people would view the first example of it only with horror. Finally, where identity in climate, productions, and diet, the same political institutions, the same domestic habits, and an equal ignorance of the agreeable arts, make it possible to establish a perfectly exact parallel between the peoples of the two communions—I mean in Switzerland— the advantage lies wholly with the Catholics, and morals were as pure in Fribourg as they were dissolute in Bern. I shall once again rest on the authority of the Bernese writer. "I know no country in Europe," he says, "where the mass of the people are less continent than in the canton of Bern"; and he cites some very strange examples of this, which recall the customs of the Lapps toward their guests, or those of the South Sea Islanders.

Moreover, it must be observed that, even given equality of disorders, the weakness of morals is more visible where it presents a greater contrast to the severity of the laws. Drunk-

*This is a compliment which the estimable Major Weiss addresses to two nations, one of which was enriching Switzerland with its guineas, while the other had accorded its protection to the canton of Bern. The most manly nations are the strongest and best, and in Europe, these are neither the English nor the Prussian.

[6] Franz Rudolph von Weiss, *Principes philosophiques, politiques et moraux, par le major Weiss* (Bern: 1785).

enness, which is not even noticed in England, is a real phenomenon in Spain; and in all countries where divorce is
allowed, it is an exceptionally good household in which
spouses do not form new ties elsewhere.

"It is in vain," says Mme. Necker, "that one seeks to
invoke, in favor of divorce, the good sense of spouses in the
Protestant countries, and the purity of domestic morals in the
first centuries of Rome. This argument appears to me worth-
less; for it only shows that the permission to divorce has no
dangerous influence in places where it is never taken advantage of." In a word, to attribute the good morals of a people to
the faculty of divorce, of which it makes no use, is to credit the
good health of a region's inhabitants to a neighboring doctor
who is never called into it.

At bottom, the goodness or corruption of marital morals lies
less in the actions which result from them than in the sentiment from which they emanate. A people given to the love of
gain, as are in general the Presbyterian peoples, is less accessible to any other sentiment. If man is good in this instance, it is
without virtue, because it is without effort; and there are no
great disorders in human affections, because there is little
affection between men. *Magis extra vitia quam cum vir-
tutibus.*[7]

But how, after all, does one dare to allege the practice of the
Protestant nations in favor of divorce, when one sees they
themselves, tired of the license it has introduced, seeking in
morals a cure for the law; Protestants themselves writing
against divorce;* and the English Parliament, convinced that
divorce today is no longer anything but a means of adultery,
occupied in preserving itself from the disastrous effects of a
law of which it was the first author?

And make no mistake: if a certain rigidity in morals, or

---

*Mme. Necker, and David Hume, Eighteenth Essay.
[7]"Rather without vices than with virtues." Tacitus, *Histories* 1.49.

rather a certain rigorism, was still visible thirty or forty years ago among the peoples who obey the Reformation, it must be attributed solely to that sectarian jealousy which, in the presence of a more severe religion, held them back on the slippery slope of corruption on which the imperfection of their dogmas places them. In this sense, the Catholic religion governed the Presbyterian religion, as Europe's monarchies governed her democracies. And one cannot doubt that morals throughout Christendom would become worse than they were under paganism, or even than they were in France at the time when vice was placed on the altars and virtue on the scaffold, if there were no other dike against their overflow than the maxims of philosophy or the phylacteries of the theophilanthropists.*

Remove Catholicism from the universe and divorce will become worse than the polygamy of the Orient, that imperfect state of domestic society, contrary to the nature of public society, which produces slavery, the exposure of children, the oppression of all the weaknesses of humanity, and is separated from the promiscuity of the beasts only by the seclusion of one sex and the mutilation of the other.

I do not fear to say it: if divorce is decreed at the same time that the exercise of the Catholic religion is established, the people will believe, either that at bottom the destruction of religion is desired, or that religion allows divorce; and either one of these opinions is capable of producing vast disorders. It can never be said often enough that divorce was only a *consequence* in 1792; one could decree anything then; the times and men provided sufficient warning against seduction. Today divorce would be seen as a *principle,* and the difference is incalculable.

I shall end with an important consideration. Marriages,

---

*These phylacteries were moral maxims which the Pharisees displayed on their chests and foreheads, and which our own theophilanthropists post on the walls of their meeting places.

which are made to unite the families of the same region, would by their dissolution become, among a sensitive and delicate people, precise appraiser of favors and insults, a fertile source of hereditary hatreds, which would return society to the age of private wars and family feuds; and there is not a single small provincial town which a single divorce could not throw into the greatest confusion. A few months ago, the *Paris Journal*[8] raised this question: *Whether the opposition in the legislature can be as vehement in France as in England.* To show that it could not, it presented reasons all of which apply far better to the question we are examining here, and maintained, on solid grounds, that among a people like the French, which *nourishes itself on bread and wine,* a personal insult does not do unpunished, nor, for far stronger reasons, does a domestic insult; for the family feud, which differs from personal vengeance, was among the Franks and is everywhere only a supplement to public prosecution, and a sure sign of the inadequacy and weakness of the political laws.

Public authority should never lose sight of the fact that religion itself, at the same time it commands man to forgive, enjoins power to punish; "for," it says, "it is not in vain that it wields the sword": *Non enim sine causa gladium portat.*[9] That is why in former times, in places where the courts could not judge and hence could not punish, public authority allowed prosecution to man in the judicial duel; and why still today, personal vengeance is more common in those countries, such as Italy, where public prosecution is less forcefully exercised. Our trial by jury in criminal matters is a remnant of the ancient domestic judgments which preceded public judgments and the regular administration of justice; a new demonstration of the rare discernment of our philosophers, who in all things are returning the most advanced nation in Europe to the imperfect customs of its earliest age.

[8] *Journal de Paris* (pub. 1777–1827).
[9] Paul, Romans 13.4.

It is therefore necessary to return to a stronger legislation, and to forbid the passions all hope of satisfying themselves legally.

It is necessary to grasp this truth, that weak laws are only suited to nascent peoples, and that laws must be more severe in proportion as society is more advanced and man looser. Thus the grown man has duties to fulfill which are far broader and involve a wholly different level of obligation than those to which the child is subject.

It is time for public power to recognize that it has trespassed on domestic power, and can reestablish good morals only by returning it its just rights, because good morals are nothing but the observation of the domestic laws. Choices will be more prudent when their consequences are more serious; power will be gentler when it is no longer contested, and when the wife has neither the property of her person nor the disposition of her goods. Peace and virtue will seat themselves at the domestic hearth when, between the father, mother, and children, the law of the State maintains the natural relationships which constitute the family, and when, in domestic as in public society, there is neither confusion of persons nor displacement of power.

CHAPTER 12

Conclusion

"LEGISLATORS, for it is to you alone that I address myself,[1] those whose heirs you are proclaimed the sovereignty of the people, and in its name they gave it political constitutions, and you yourselves give it civil laws. But has the French nation given you, has it even been able to give you, the power to denature its domestic constitution, unshakeable foundation of the edifice it has inhabited for so many centuries? Can you have believed that the fathers of families, convened in the primary assemblies, have agreed to abdicate domestic power into your hands, so that their wives may receive power from the law to rise against them, dispute their actions, drag them before the courts, and present their depositions, in order to transfer marital authority to other hands, or to remove their children from paternal authority? No, the French people has not forgotten nature, reason, and its dignity to such a point; and if you doubt this, observe with what resounding marks of disapproval it rejects in the theater* this law which is the

---

*At the performance of the play the *Amiable Elder*, which the audience did not wish to be completed. Yet the proposition of divorce in it was only simulated.[2]

[1] The concluding chapter of the work is cast as a speech. The ellipses in it indicate pauses, not missing text. The "legislators" Bonald is addressing would have been the members of the Council of State, which began discussion of the proposed Civil Code on 4 Thermidor, Year IX (July 23, 1801). In the event, Bonald incorporated large sections of this chapter into the crucial speech he gave in the Chamber of Deputies in 1815. Louis de Bonald, *Proposition faite à la Chambre des députés, séance du 26 décembre 1815*, 24 pp. (Paris: Hacquart, n.d.).

[2] Augustin Prévost, *L'aimable vieillard* (Paris: Perreault, 1803). In the preface to the play, the author protests that "I shall leave behind me no evidence of

object of the public authorities' most serious deliberations; and you yourselves, legislators, did you not brand it at its birth with the mark of infamy, and will it not be said, concerning the difficulties with which you surround its execution, that you permit divorce only on condition that we never make use of it?

"A part of the nation, you say, professes a religion which tolerates divorce.* . . . But do you count for nothing the entire nation, which professes a religion which forbids it? And if you think you should not deprive a few of what is for them only a mere possibility, why do you allow the greatest number what they regard as a crime?

"You grant divorce, because a part of the nation professes a religion which tolerates its faculty; . . . but would you allow theft to the votaries of a religion (and there have been such) which established as a principle the community of goods?

"You respect the faculty of divorce as a toleration of the Protestant religion, and you do not respect separation, which is a toleration of the Catholic religion! You allow some the rupture of the conjugal tie, too often solicited by mad passions or vile interests, and you forbid the others all loosening of it, which is often necessary to forestall worse explosions, and sometimes the ultimate misfortunes! and you place those citizens who are most attached to the severe maxims of their belief in a position beyond the strength of man, because it is contrary to reason, between two contradictory powers which are equally imperious!†

"But at bottom there is not, even on this question, between the two parties which your imprudent law restores to life, as much opposition as you suppose.

---

misconduct nor any writing which can show my immorality or has ever denigrated anyone." Prévost was also the author of a play called *L'utilité du divorce* ("The Utility of Divorce").

*Since the expansion of France, and according to the latest censuses, Protestants of both communions represent about one-fortieth of the total population.

†The Civil Code has admitted separation.

"The principle of the natural indissolubility of the conjugal tie is universally received by all Christian communions; and not only do the reformed communions acknowledge it in speculation, but they follow it in practice, since wherever the weakness of their doctrine is contained by the presence of a more severe doctrine, they make use of divorce only rarely, even in France formerly, although their marriages, far from being guaranteed by the law there, were not even recognized by the legislator. But the Protestants differ from the Catholics on the question of marriage, in that the Protestants believe its indissolubility to be natural, and do not believe it to be religious, whereas the Catholics believe indissolubility to be religious, because it is perfect or natural, and was so *in the beginning.* They believe that there is nothing more religious than what is natural or good; that man cannot dissolve what nature, and therefore its author, has united; for that is the meaning of this passage: *Quod Deus conjunxit, homo non separet;*[3] and that the universal legislator, whose divine wisdom is acknowledged by all Christian communions, *come,* he himself says, *to accomplish the law,* that is to say, to perfect it by conforming it in all ways to the nature of beings, can have allowed nothing contrary to nature. The authors of the proposed Civil Code themselves establish the principle of the indissolubility of the conjugal tie, when they say: 'Marriage, considered in itself and in its *natural relationships,* presents the fundamental idea of a contract perpetual in its goal, and the wish of perpetuity in marriage appears to be the very wish of nature'; and nevertheless they reach a conclusion against the principle of the Catholics, against the principle of the Protestants, against their own principle, against nature, against reason, which says that what is indissoluble by nature cannot be dissolved by man; they violate the conscience of the greater number, in order to let the conscience of the lesser enjoy a simple toleration; they induce some to become guilty, out of

[3] "What God has joined together, let not man put asunder." Matthew 19.6.

Conclusion 133

fear of obliging others to be consistent; and they weaken the
strong, when one should assist and encourage the weak.

"You do not wish to interfere with religious beliefs. . . . If
you enjoin the Protestants to believe in the *Real Presence,* or
the Catholics to believe in the *inamissibility of justice,* you will
interfere with religious beliefs; but then you will not be
obeyed, because beliefs, religious or political, are outside of
your competence. But divorce is not a belief, but a social
action, that is to say, domestic in its principle, public in its
effects, like marriage and like man himself; an action which
religion prescribes or forbids, like all social actions; for note
that separation, which it merely allows, is not a social action,
since it does not lead to any new state of society; now, you
claim to have the right to permit, to forbid, to regulate social
actions, even religious ones, which, exercised outside the
precincts of the temples, enter the category of civil acts. Thus
you have changed the fundamental law of religious worship,
which consecrates the seventh day to physical rest, by com-
manding public work on that day, or by allowing domestic
work, and fixing the weekly rest on the tenth day;* thus you
forbid ceremonies of worship and religious vestments outside
the temples, actions which are good in themselves, or at least
indifferent; and you seem to believe that a divorce is less
external than a procession, or less of an assault on authority
than a long robe. You respect in divorce a religious belief . . . ;
but you would not allow Chinese living in France, and permitted, by your laws, to practice their religion there, to sacrifice
their children to the *spirit of the river* by drowning them, even
in their temples; Indian widows to burn themselves on the
bodies of their husbands; or Turks to maintain *harems* in the
middle of Paris, although their religious beliefs permit or pre-

*The law of Sunday prescribes the suspension of physical and domestic
activity only in order that man may participate in religious activity or
worship. *Decadi,* in contrast, is a day of absolute rest, and nothing in nature,
except for God alone, rests. See in a little work, written by a very learned
man, and published by Didot, the natural reasons for the old division of time.

scribe all of these actions. Will you say that infanticide is more contrary to nature than mutual divorce, or the repudiation of the husband by the wife? Infanticide destroys man; divorce dissolves society. The child is not naturally immortal; marriage is naturally indissoluble. The exposure of children does not produce divorce; divorce produces the neglect of children, and often compromises their lives. Morals in Rome resisted the atrocious law of infanticide, practiced since the earliest times, but they could not resist the frequent practice of divorce, which began at the end of the republic, because infanticide is the abuse of paternal authority, while divorce is the annihilation of domestic power.

"You do not wish to interfere with religious beliefs. . . . But is it the belief in the faculty of divorce, or the belief in the indissolubility of the conjugal tie, which is a religious belief? I see what is religious in believing that society, instituted by God against human passions, cannot be dissolved by man, and upon his whims; that marriage, which must be the cure for voluptuousness, would be only its spur and means, if the faculty of divorce ceaselessly delivered new objects to man's desires; and that the father of humans has not established a society among his children where the weak being, unconditionally delivered to the stronger, fails to find, against her own passions, a perpetual protection in exchange for an irrevocable sacrifice. Outside of this, I am far from seeing religious beliefs, and I do not even see reasonable ones.

"Beware: divorce can only be a religious toleration for those who see a religious bond in marriage, and who, like the Jews, allow its dissolution by the same authority which has established it. But how can it be a religious faculty for those who see nothing sacred in the institution? By what inconsistency can one consider the faculty of divorce a dogma, when one does not consider marriage a sacrament? and how can a civil law, given by Solon to an idolatrous people, be a religious faculty given by Jesus Christ to Christians?

"But, after all, the Christian religion tolerates nothing; neither evil, since it forbids it; nor good, since it commands it. It tolerates only perfection, which is to say that it recommends it; and far from tolerating divorce, which gives man the faculty to dismiss his neighbor's daughter, and marry his neighbor's wife, it allows the faculty of celibacy, by allowing man to devote himself to the ministry of religious society. And there are no grounds for astonishment at this, nor, as our philosophers have done, to take it as an opportunity to declaim against religion, since one sees political society, forced to employ in its service the entire youth of a nation, making celibacy indispensable for it, and even condemning the greater number to a premature death, before having tasted the delights of marriage.

"It is time to say it: divorce is a purely human opinion; and surely, when all parties were agreed on the natural indissolubility of the conjugal tie, there was little philosophy in concluding that it could be humanly dissolved. That is nevertheless the conclusion which the sixteenth-century reformers drew; but at bottom, legislators, who have yourselves come to reform a great nation, were their rights to reform greater than yours? Their partisans today attribute no divine mission to them, and they had not, like you, been sent by electoral assemblies; or if one wishes, today as in their time, to regard the rapid propagation of their doctrine as a miracle which proves the truth of their mission, what advantage would you not have over them, even in this regard? Luther, in the sixteenth century, swayed Germans and Swiss, and you, in the nineteenth century, have made yourselves obeyed by the French.*

---

*The followers of Luther regarded the rapid progress of his doctrine as a miracle which proved his mission; and certainly, it is true that Luther's opinions made considerably more of a stir at their birth than the doctrine of the gospel itself. Some opinions explode like volcanoes, and sweep along everything in their path like floods swollen by the storm; others gain ground little by little, by an insensible progress, *like dough which ferments,* or like *the seed* which takes root before raising itself and *becoming a great tree.*

"More enlightened today by the progress of time and enlightenment, and stronger by virtue of the means you control, dare* to reform the reformers themselves: so many others have done it since they appeared. Do not speak in the name of the Catholic Church, you will not be believed; speak in the name of nature and reason, and you will be listened to. What am I saying! the reformers themselves would reform their principles today, and would judge that in the nineteenth century, the century of riches and arts, divorce must produce far more unhappy effects than in the sixteenth century, when there were as yet neither large cities, nor commerce, theaters, public promenades, statues, or novels, when spouses knew only their hearths, and citizens no other public places than the town hall and the church; and do we not already see their descendants, tired of the intolerable yoke of license, rising up against the faculty of divorce, and the English Parliament deliberating on its inadequacy? Listen to Mme. Necker, as attached as she is to the Calvinist religion, concurring on this point with the doctrine of the Catholic Church.

Before criticizing (she says) the fathers of the Church, who raised marriage to the rank of a sacrament, one must know the principle of their decision. A little reflection will persuade us that *nothing was more in accordance* with what was required, with the laws and rights of nature: for to make marriage a merely civil contract is to take, as the basis for this institution, the least important circumstance. And indeed, fortune, the State, all the formalities of the civil sphere, are simple accessories in a commitment whose purpose is the association of hearts, sentiments, reputations, and lives; and since all great affections have constantly been joined to religious ideas, since, in society, oaths cement all commitments which the law is

---

*Deliberation alone, to find out whether divorce should be introduced or rejected, is a mortal blow against the Protestant religion, as it is against the Catholic religion; for if it was possible to introduce divorce against the principles of the one, it is possible to reject it against the opinions of the other.

unable to supervise, why except marriage from this general rule, marriage, the perfect purity of which can have no other judge or witness than our own conscience? "The exclusion of polygamy and divorces," says M. Hume (Eighteenth Essay), "sufficiently recommends our present European practice with regard to marriage."

"At this point inconsistencies multiply: the Civil Code proposes divorce, because of the Lutherans and the Protestants, and it proposes it neither like Luther nor like Calvin. In effect, Luther, in his first work, *On the Babylonian Captivity,*[4] desires that the conjugal tie be subject to dissolution for the cause of adultery or malicious desertion; but, still timid, he does not dare to proclaim it dissolved. Three years later, having doubtless become more clever or less restrained, he allows divorce on these two grounds, and even on several others. Melancthon, the most learned of his disciples, reduces the grounds to two, adultery and desertion. Calvin dissolves the conjugal tie for the cause of adultery, or when one of the parties, being Christian, wishes to separate from the idolatrous party; so that, leaving aside the variations of the heads and the extravagances of a few disciples, and among others *Bucer,* who allowed divorce for the slightest discontent, the reformed of all sects agree on this sole point, that the conjugal tie is dissolved for the cause of adultery and desertion.

"The legislators of '92 came in their turn; they raised the stakes on those who had come before, by decreeing divorce for incompatibility of temperament; and even the authors of the proposed Civil Code declare the request for divorce to be admissible *for offenses and crimes of one spouse against the other,* that is to say, as the proposal explains: (1) *for cruelty and ill-treatment, and habitual conduct of one spouse toward the other which renders life unbearable for the latter;* (2) *by public defamation;* (3) *by desertion of the husband by the wife,*

[4] Martin Luther, *De Captivitate Babylonica Ecclesiae* (Strasbourg: J. Prüss, 1520).

or of the wife by the husband; (4) *by the attempted murder of one spouse by the other;* (5) finally, and as a postscript, *by the adultery of the wife, accompanied by a public scandal, and proven by writings emanating from her, and by that of the husband who keeps his concubine in the common household.* So that, out of all the grounds for divorce, the most common and at the same time the most legitimate, the only one which is authorized by the gospel, according to Protestants, and which gives rise, according to Catholics, to the request for separation, adultery, is precisely the one which it will henceforth be impossible to prove: for women are well warned by this law that they can allow everything to their weakness, except to write their lovers; men, that they can allow everything to their passions, except to house the concubine under the same roof as the wife; and short of a solemn prostitution in the public square, how is it possible to prove any *public scandal* where the extreme easiness of morals permits all frivolities, and knows almost no further inconsequence? And certainly one cannot help noticing what a terrible oppression will weigh on the wife, whose condition and honor will henceforth depend on a writing, at a time when the art of altering, removing, and counterfeiting handwriting has been carried to such a deplorable degree of perfection.*

"Admire nonetheless the progress of certain doctrines, and how man, once he has left the narrow path of truth, strays in proportion as he advances on the infinite roads of error, and can only find rest by returning to his starting point. Thanks to the strength of our laws, and in spite of the frivolity of our morals, the forms of marriage were more severe in France, and its effects much better ensured, in our time than formerly. The requirement for the presence of the personal pastor for the validity of marriages forestalled clandestine unions; the re-

---

*The court of Mainz has just pronounced a divorce between the count and countess of Leiningen-Guntersblum, who have had several children together, for an *insulting letter* written by the husband to the wife.

quirement for the consent of the parents prevented rash commitments; and bastardy itself, in spite of philosophy, was day
by day becoming more disgraceful. And indeed, in the upper
classes of society, divorce, tolerated by the constitutions of the
Greek emperors, and repudiation, occasionally practiced by
the Franks, had disappeared from our laws and morals, and
Christianity had been working for fifteen centuries to lead man
to the perfection of maturity, by giving him a more correct
conception of his duties, made sensible by a more decent
expression in discourse: and here, in less than three centuries,
a purely human wisdom, sometimes under one name, sometimes under another, has made society retrogress all the way to
the imperfect customs of the earliest age, and has thrown it
back even further than the barbarism of the most savage state;
as if moral beings in their progress were subject to laws like
those of heavy bodies in their movements, as delayed in their
ascent as they are accelerated in their fall.

"In effect, before Luther and Calvin, there were passions
among men, as there have been since, as there will always be;
but there were, in the Christian world, neither divorces nor
separations; and indeed it was not far from the time when the
Popes contained the peoples, still crude and little enlightened,
by great examples, and smote with their censure kings who
contracted illegitimate ties or broke solemn ones. Scarcely had
the Reformation opened the door of divorce to the passions
than they rushed to it like a crowd, *qua data porta ruunt;*[5] and
when divorces began among the Protestants, the practice and
soon the abuse of separations began among the Catholics,
and continuously increased. Philosophy appeared at the end of
time, and not only, like the heads of the Reformation, did it
allow the dissolution of the conjugal tie, but it allowed it with
all the variants of their disciples; to which it added its own,
and allowed divorce for all sorts of causes, and even *for*

[5] "Once the door is opened, they rush in."

incompatibility of temperament; or, what amounts to about the same thing, *for habitual conduct which makes life in common unbearable*. For what cannot be included under this vague expression, now that with the distaste for domestic pleasures, caused by the profusion of public ones, or by the excess of clandestine ones, so many men and women, consumed by disgust and boredom, far from being able mutually to endure each other, blasé toward all pleasures, and even toward life itself, can no longer endure themselves? Divorce is allowed for motives such that no contract in civil life would be possible if it could be terminated on such vague pretexts. One more legislature, and we shall fall into the community of women and the promiscuity of the beasts; for the weakness of marital authority will not allow us to stop at the polygamy of the Orientals. Future legislators will possess, to justify the community of the sexes, the grounds which past and present legislators have possessed to advocate such a broad faculty of divorce; and if the latter have been motivated by the frequency of separations, the former will excuse themselves by the multiplicity of concubinages. For do not doubt, legislators, already people contract less, and soon they will not contract at all bonds degraded by the extreme ease of breaking them. 'At the time when divorces were most frequent among the Romans,' says Hume in his *Essays,* 'marriages were most rare; and Augustus was obliged, by penal laws, to force the citizens into the married state.'[6] And what interest could make a man endure the cares and trials of domesticity, in a country where the man with a wife and children is never sure, thanks to the faculty of divorce, that he will continue to have a family?

"Thus, in the course of three centuries in which a human

[6] Hume does not say "the citizens" but "men of fashion." Bonald was presumably working from the eighteenth-century French translation of Hume's *Essays,* which translates "men of fashion" literally, producing an unintelligible phrase, *gens de façon*. Cf. David Hume, *Essais moraux et politiques,* in *Oeuvres de M. D. Hume,* translated by J. B. Merian, 6 vols. (London: David Wilson, 1764), vol. 6, p. 226.

philosophy has dictated laws to Europe, it has given her divorce, demagogy, and indifferentism to all religion. France, its latest conquest, has borne the weight of its scorn and pride; vile subject of all experiments, toy of all its whims, she has received from it the period of the *Terror*, the reign of the *sansculottes*, the doctrines of Chaumette and Marat, the tyranny of Robespierre, the cult of the goddess Reason; and she could apply to herself what Tacitus so energetically says of the Britons, last to fall under Roman domination: '*In hoc orbis terrarum vetere famulatu novi nos et viles in excidium petimur.*'[7]

"Thus man's morals are corrupted in proportion as society's laws are weakened, and the laws are weakened in proportion as morals are corrupted; thus the laws have served as a spur to man's desires, once they no longer served as a bridle on his passions. And do not present the frequency of separations as evidence of the need for divorce. Legislators, know human nature and its penchants: if today you decree that children may repulse their fathers' outbursts of temper by force, tomorrow you will be surrounded by parricides.

"The law, you say, allows divorce; but, far from requiring it, hinders its faculty. But is it a question of making divorce difficult, or of making marriage honorable? Will the passions, which strive today against the law of indissolubility, respect the barriers surrounding divorce? And if there were only, as among the Romans, a single example of it after several centuries, is French legislation any less dishonored in its principle, and the French nation less weakened in its laws? The law does not require divorce. . . . Legislators, among a people little advanced in the arts, the toleration of divorce is without danger, because it is without example. In that age of society, man sees in woman only the mother of his children and the governess of his house. His love for her is esteem, and the

---

[7] "In a world long used to slavery, we, as the newest and vilest of slaves, are singled out for destruction." Tacitus, *Agricola* 31.2.

woman's love for her husband is respect. Virginity, chastity are
honored; and all the refinements of sensibility, which present
one sex to the other in terms of personal pleasure and senti-
mental affection, are unknown to their simplicity. But when a
society has reached the point that the mad loves of youth,
inexhaustible element of the arts, have become, under a thousand forms, the talk of all ages; when marital authority is a
derision, and paternal authority a tyranny; when obscene
books, displayed everywhere, sold or rented so cheaply one
would think they were given away, reveal to the child what
nature does not teach even the grown man, and the whole
panoply of learning and the whole perfection of art are used to
transmit to us the history of the vices of Greece,* after having
spoken to us so often of the novel of its virtues, in order to
corrupt us both by the morals of its prostitutes and the laws of
its sages; when man's nudity, distinctive trait of extreme bar-
barity, presents itself to our view on all sides in public places,
and woman herself, clothed without being concealed, has discovered the art of insulting modesty without shocking propriety; when between men there are only physical differences,
and no social distinctions, and in place of those respectful
designations which make the sexes disappear beneath the
dignity of expressions we are all—shall I say it?—just males
and females; when religion has lost all its terrors, and philosopher spouses see in their reciprocal infidelities only a
secret to be mutually hushed, or possibly a confidence to
make each other: then to tolerate divorce is to command
prostitution and legalize adultery; it is to conspire with man's
passions against his reason, and with man himself against
society. After this, establish funds to reward the virtue of
maidens; write idylls to proclaim the happiness of marriage;

---

*The scandalous history of the *Courtesans of Greece* was published at the
same time as the first edition of this work. Fortunately its stupidity dimin-
ishes its danger.[8]
[8] *Les courtisanes de la Grèce* (Paris: Gay et Gide, Year II [1793]).

offer bounties for fertility, and levy taxes on celibacy, and you will see, with all these philosophical means, the disorders of voluptuousness increase along with the distaste for marriage, and our morals become, if possible, as weak as your laws. France's territory has increased; but her dignity, the first means of her might, founded on the decency of her morals and the severity of her laws, has been eclipsed. Where foreigners were unable to breach her frontiers, her own children have ruined the family, religion, and the State, with the license of divorce, of philosophism, and of demagogy. Moral man has disappeared; and like those rivers which vanish in the sand, useless for cultivation when no dike restrains them, his soul has no more resilience, because his desires have no more stopping point. Those violent passions, tumultuous storm of the human heart, those terrible battles of love against duty, of the most impetuous of sentiments against the mightiest of obstacles, which honor human nature even when it succumbs, and whose fiction excites so much admiration and moves us to so many tears, would no longer be anything but chimeras, which a degenerate posterity will relegate to the rank of the labors of Hercules or the war of the gods and the Titans. Legislators, close these theaters, which have for so long been the ornament of France. Phèdre, Zénobie, Pauline, Monime would be inconceivable characters for a nation which knows divorce. Andromache,* reduced to saving her son's life by betraying the faith she had promised her first husband, and swearing to die while forming new bonds, would excite only ridicule from women able to remarry even while their husbands are still living. These great scenes of society, in which man appears in all his strength, because duty shows itself in all its rigor, and virtue in all its austerity, would no longer be credible as dramatic subjects; and since this childish people

---

*"One does not believe," says Racine in the preface to *Andromache*, "that she should love a husband other than Hector, or children other than those she had by him."

must have spectacles, its idleness will be entertained by lack-eys' antics,* harlequin farces, and ghost and crime stories.

"Vows to remain united forever, sacred commitments which love and innocence believe to be eternal, you are no illusion! nature inspires you in all hearts taken with each other; but, stronger than nature, and in accord with her against our passions, a sacred and sublime law had ratified you; and halting forever man's heart at these sentiments, so pure and, alas! so fugitive, it had given our weakness the divine character of its immutability. And here is the legislator of divorce, who has hoped in our inconstancy, and abused the secret of our penchants. His sad and cruel foresight has come to alert the heart of its disgusts, and the passions of their dominion. Like the slaves who were included in the triumph of conquerors, to remind them that they were men, it comes, but with a very different purpose, to shout at virtue, on the most sacred days of its joy, that it is weak and changeable, not to fortify, but to corrupt it; not to promise its support, but to offer its criminal complaisances. At the very moment that the spouses are swearing eternal fidelity, that religion is consecrating their vows, that their deeply moved families are breaking into applause, a fatal law secretly pours its poison into the cup of union, and hides a viper under the flowers. It makes the ears of the couple ring with the words of separation and divorce, and leaves in the heart, like a mortal blow, the doubt of its own constancy, and the possibility of a happier attempt.

"And yet a mother had led a beloved daughter to the altar; intoxicated with maternal joy, she projected the sweet hopes of tenderness into the future, and saw in the object of her affections a happy woman and an honored wife. The unfortunate did not foresee that one day her daughter, dismissed without

---

*The limited ideas of the people have never been so ridiculed in the theater as since it has been acknowledged sovereign. These depictions spoil the well brought up without correcting the lower classes, whose domestic *simpleness* must be respected, and their political rights not exaggerated.

honor from her husband's house, and fleeing before a haughty rival, would return to water the paternal doorstep with the tears of despair, and reproach her parents for choosing a deceiver; or that perhaps, having become guilty herself through the seduction of the law, she would seek in shame a refuge from misery, and escape disgrace only through impudence.

"Divorce is said to increase population, but what is not realized is that if the union of the sexes populates an uninhabited country, only the society of the spouses maintains and increases the population of an established nation, and that divorce, where the legislator has the imprudence to introduce or conserve its faculty, kills more families than it engenders children. The savages' little tribes, where all individuals marry, are weak and miserable; and among civilized peoples, where the needs of society condemn a large part of the nation to celibacy, the State is populous and flourishing. One pities spouses whom simple separation condemns to an austere solitude; but is it for legislators to attend to the pleasures of the individual at the expense of society? Does one expect to remedy all the disorders of incontinence with the faculty of divorce? and does one not know that an absolute chastity is less painful to man than a severe temperance?

> Divorce for infidelity (says Mme. Necker) stigmatizes the guilty party and afflicts the offended one; but the perjurer can no more be allowed to form new bonds than an outlaw to return to the country where he was condemned; and as for the husband or wife who has been outraged, the lot has fallen to them to offer a great example of delicacy. They will weep in the desert like Jephthah's daughter; but like her they will live alone, out of respect for vows uttered in the presence of heaven. Many people have destined themselves to celibacy who have not had such pure and respectable motives.

"You reproach the law of indissolubility with its perfection, and the only question is our perfectibility; you charge this law

with impracticability, and it is practiced almost everywhere, at
least *de facto;* for even where divorce is allowed, it is always
rarer than undissolved marriages. But see too the sophists,
who accuse of severity the law which punishes homicide with
death. A strange inconsistency! the deists find man too vile for
the Supreme Being to deign to lower himself to him; Jean-
Jacques Rousseau finds man too dull to be taught, before the
age of fifteen, that he has a soul; modern legislators find man
too imperfect for them to be able to give him strong laws: and
yet they make of man, they make of the people, the infallible
legislator, the universal sovereign; and from so many imperfections in the parts, they assemble perfection itself in the
whole. The law of indissolubility is too perfect! Well, what
about it? The legislator of the Christians, in the midst of all the
pagan voluptuosities and all the Judaic crudities, told men: *Be
perfect;* and immediately they cast out of society all those
imperfect or corrupt laws of their childhood: slavery, polygamy, atrocious and licentious spectacles, divination, the sacrifice of human victims, the immolation of animals, etc., etc.
Still today men, saying he has sent them, plant a wooden cross
in the desert, and, ministers of this new authority, change the
customs of ancient times in a day; order the naked man to
clothe himself, the wandering man to settle down, the hunter
to cultivate the earth, the polygamist to unite with his fellow
being by an indissoluble bond, the idolator to worship one
God alone, creator and conservator: and they are obeyed; and
refinement begins with Christianity; and the comforts of life
along with the duties of society; and the *culture* of the useful
arts along with the *cult* of God; and such is the strength of this
severe doctrine, all the more natural to man's reason as it is
opposed to his penchants, that thousands of Christians, whose
minds were as just as their hearts were upright, have suffered,
to remain faithful to these beliefs which according to you are
unbelievable, from these practices which you accuse of impracticability, hurts and torments which philosophy would not

endure to maintain its facile doctrine and conserve its licentious morals. And you, legislators, after man, having left weakness and childhood behind him, has attained, with the help of Christianity, *the measure of the age* of maturity, and the *fullness* of social *perfection, virum perfectum in mensuram aetatis plenitudinis Christi,*[9] you wish to make him redescend to the puerilities of the earliest age, and to put back on the milk of infancy men accustomed to the substantial nourishment of the Christian religion. 'Vain and false philosophy,' exclaims Saint Paul, 'which would return the world to the elements of its childhood, and make it fall from the dignity of Christianity!' *Videte ne quis vos decipiat per philosophiam, et inanem fallaciam, secundum elementa mundi et non secundum Christum.*[10]

"The world will therefore see something it has never seen: legislators proposing weak laws to peoples accustomed to strong ones, and who claim them as their property; it will see sages less wise than the vulgar, the forum more grave than the Senate, and the theater more austere than the Stoa. For the French people, even in the most obscure classes, rejects the faculty of divorce with horror, and its good sense, which philosophical doctrines have nowise altered, makes it perceive this faculty's injustice and danger.

"Legislators, it tells you, why should men today be beneath the perfection of the laws, since they know it better than ever, and have for so long made it the rule of their conduct? Has there been some change in human nature? Is the Frenchman less enlightened, after a century of enlightenment, or less strong, after the days of his conquests? You want to make us better, and you begin by allowing us to be wicked; you trace us

[9] "A man perfect in the measure of the age of the fullness of Christ." Paul, Ephesians 4.13.
[10] "See to it that no one deceives you through philosophy and empty trickery according to the elements of the world and not according to Christ." Paul, Colossians 2.8.

rules, and they are less upright than our penchants. What are we supposed to do with a support which cannot sustain us? You tell us you have consulted our morals, and you have only taken counsel with our passions; you have made laws for voluptuousness and inconstancy; *you have darkened the eye, which should light up the rest of the body,* and falsified the rule, so as to make rectification impossible.

"The authors of the proposed Civil Code *have seen,* they say, *the action of time and the march of events,* and all they have seen is the action of man and the march of his passions. Man deteriorates, but time perfects, because time discovers truth; and instead of *enchaining* the action of time, as they put it, one should assist the action of time and enchain that of man. They have seen a few men practicing divorce, and they have not seen society expelling it from the very nations where it has long been practiced, and which, internally perturbed by this principle of death, will only find peace by returning to the order which they have abandoned. *For,* your oracle tells you, *if the legislator, mistaking his object, establishes a principle different from that which arises from the nature of things, the State will not cease to be agitated until it is destroyed or changed, and invincible nature has resumed her sway. (Social Contract.)*

"Let us benefit from this wise lesson; let us dare to think like rational beings, and to say like free men: that the State has power over the family only to strengthen its ties, not to dissolve them; and that if the State destroys the family, the family in turn avenges itself and quietly undermines the State. Alas! we do not dispute the government's terrible but necessary power to annihilate our families, by sacrificing in its defense those whom nature had destined to perpetuate them, and whom we had raised with a different hope; but we dispute its right to corrupt them, by destroying authority in the husband, subordination in the wife, dependence in the child, and by failing to leave us, against public depravity, the refuge of the domestic virtues; and, since it must be said, the peoples have been told only too much about their duty to demand their rights, and have perhaps never been told of their duty to defend their virtues.

"Legislators, you have seen divorce produce demagogy, and the *deconstitution* of the family precede that of the State. May this experience be lost neither for your instruction nor for our happiness. The family requires morals, and the State requires laws. Strengthen domestic power, natural element of public power, and consecrate the complete dependence of children, guarantee of the continual obedience of peoples. Take care not to create powers where nature has placed only duties, by decreeing the civil equality of persons distinguished from one another by domestic inequalities. Condemned to rebuild the edifice, since you are the heirs of those who destroyed it, and free to coordinate all its parts according to a regular plan, leave nothing vicious in it, if you cannot banish all imperfection. A wise government arranges everything for the good, even when it cannot do everything for the best; and divorce is not a gap to fill, as the proposed Code says, it is a canker to extirpate.

"For the past ten years, men in France have been making laws as weak and transient as they themselves; declare at last those eternal laws which men *do not make,** but which make men. It is not on the basis of fundamental laws, which are the principles of all subsequent and statutory ones, that *it is absurd to give oneself up to absolute ideas of perfection;* because the goodness of these laws is absolute, and they EMANATE directly *from the supreme reason, from the universal reason,* which is essentially perfect. Command us to be good, and we will be so. Make Europe forget her disorders by force of wisdom, as you have erased our shame by force of success. You have made France the great nation by her ex-

---

*Introduction to the proposed Civil Code, from which is also taken that which is emphasized in the following lines.

ploits, make her the good nation by her morals and her laws. We have enough glory, and too many pleasures; it is time to give us virtues. Reflect that the age which society has reached no longer allows the weak laws and soft complaisances appropriate only to its childhood: sorrow and shame on the government that would make social man retrogress toward the imperfection of the earliest age; it will found the social edifice on the shifting sands of human passions; and it will sow disorder, and leave the following generations with revolutions to reap."

APPENDIX

APPENDIX

I.

Excerpt from
the *Harmony of Revelation and Reason against Divorce,*
by M. l'abbé de Chapt de Rastignac[1]

The Church of Poland

Around 1549, Sigismund Augustus II, king of Poland, had just married Barbara Radziwill; the conditions of the spouses were utterly disproportionate. In the diet held at Piotrków that same year, the Poles pressed him to break the marriage, because the king had married without consulting the Senate, and one of the laws of Poland was that the king could not contract an alliance with anyone without consulting it. On this occasion, the Poles extended to marriage something that only concerned treaties with foreign princes. The prince resisted them, opposing to them the indissolubility of marriage, although the Archbishop of Gniezno protested to him, in his own name and in that of the entire diet, that they would all take the sin on themselves in the event that there had been one. The king stood firm: would Augustus II have been able to oppose

---

[1] The text that follows through page 160 is reproduced verbatim, including quotations and footnotes, from *L'accord de la Révélation et de la Raison contre le divorce,* by the abbé Armand de Chapt de Rastignac (Paris: Clousier, 1790), pp. 247–259. Rastignac's book is an erudite polemic against Albert-Joseph-Ulpien Hennet's *Du divorce* ("On Divorce"; Paris: Desenne, 1789), a work in favor of divorce addressed to the Constituent Assembly. It seems possible that the title of Bonald's book, *On Divorce, Considered in the Nineteenth Century,* was intended as a riposte to Hennet's *On Divorce.*

the indissolubility of marriage to the Poles if divorce had been allowed in Poland?*

Pope Pius V exhorted this prince not to break his marriage in any way. He wrote to the king:

> You should be aware that those who, under pretext of assuring the hoped-for succession, are attempting to convince you to do a thing of this nature are either heretics or inciters of heretics, and have nothing more at heart than to engage you to pass, at least once, beyond the bounds of Catholic truth, convinced that if they can obtain this from you by a crime, or rather extort it, the rest will be easier for them.†

If the Catholic Church in Poland had allowed divorce, would the Pope have characterized as heretics or inciters of heretics those who counseled Augustus II to break his marriage?

Cardinal Hosius, bishop of Varmia, one of the presidents of the Council of Trent under Pius IV, and one of the greatest men of his time, of whom the Emperor Ferdinand said that his mouth was a temple and his tongue an oracle of the Holy Spirit, clearly teaches the indissolubility of marriage.

> Let marriage (he says) not be separated, and let the dismissed spouse not unite himself with another to have children; for this is the word of the Lord: *I tell you that whoever divorces his wife, except for the cause of fornication, causes her to commit adultery;* and furthermore: *What God has joined together, let not man put asunder.* And Saint Paul, following his master, tells those who are married: "I command, yet not I, but the Lord, that a wife must not separate herself from her husband; if she does, she must either remain unmarried or be reconciled to her husband." These words of Jesus Christ and of the apostle were understood no differently by Saint Ambrose, Saint Jerome, Saint Augustine, and before them, neither by Origen, nor by

---

Art of Verif. Dates, vol. 2, p. 73.[2]
†*Pius V,* bk. 5, epist. 1.
[2] Dom Maur-François Dantine et al., *Art de vérifier les dates,* 3d ed., 3 vols. (Paris: Alexandre Jombert jeune, 1783–1787; orig. ed. 1750).

Saint Chrysostom, nor by Theophylactus, who follows in his footsteps, nor the other holy doctors. . . . The case of the man is no different, and it should not involve more favorable conditions than that of the woman.*

Flagrant abuses with regard to marriage had introduced themselves into Poland. In order to remedy these, Benedict XIV sent instructions to the bishops of Poland in 1741. In November of the same year, he issued a ruling on the manner of judging marriage cases. He decreed that sentences of annulment could be appealed. The Poles had made agreements not to appeal such sentences. On April 1, 1743, the Pope issued a new bull which, "in providing for the stability of marriages, condemns or annuls the agreements made between spouses not to appeal sentences of *annulment* of marriage."

After having exposed the abuse, Benedict XIV indicated its causes:

> We are convinced (he says) that the disorder and confusion of which we have spoken above, and which reign in the kingdom of Poland, come, for the most part, from the manner in which marriages are contracted and celebrated there: very often the parties' own parish priest does not participate in them; sometimes, without his knowledge, the commission is given to any priest whatever to participate; very often, too, the publication of banns is dispensed with, so that, even though there is no legitimate and pressing cause, not a single bann is published. By this one closes every route through which it would have been possible to know whether the marriage was celebrated with the necessary freedom on the part of both the contracting parties, and their consent; if there is no impediment between the two, by reason of which the same marriage, once contracted, would have to be subsequently dissolved and begun over. This gives rise to frequent disputes over the annulment of marriages, even though they were celebrated within the Church. Sometimes it is claimed that the marriage was contracted either through vio-

*Stanisl. Hosii opera, edit. in-fol. Colon. 1584.

lence or through fear, without the free consent of one of the two spouses. Sometimes an impediment is produced which, although legitimate and canonical, could have been discovered before the marriage was contracted, if it had not been expressly and intentionally intended that it remain hidden. On other occasions, and this occurs more frequently, the annulment of the marriage is based on its having been celebrated in front of a different priest by a commission, either of the vicar or of the bishop, which was not given according to the required and customary forms: certainly, there is no one who does not sense that, all this providing an easy entry to crime, is cause that the canonical favor of appeal which we have granted in our most recent letters, which one of the spouses may enjoy following the sentence he has obtained concerning the nullity of the marriage, is interfered with by these frauds and subterfuges, and that dissolutions of marriage are very frequent in Poland, to the very great scandal of good people.*

These dissolutions of marriage are thus not founded in Poland on the faculty of divorce, but on grounds for annulment and diriment impediments.

The custom of Poland (says the author of the *Matrimonial Code*), far from establishing that divorce is authorized there, demonstrates the contrary. When a marriage contracted by violence is dissolved, it is because it is judged that there was never any consent, and that as consent is at the basis of marriage as of any contract, it is judged that there was never any marriage; as soon as one finds no other means to enable two spouses tired of each other's society to form a new one, than to declare that there was never any commitment to connect them, it is a sensible proof that if there had been a commitment, it could only have been indissoluble; after this, although judges may be more or less ready to admit evidence of this nullity of commitment, the law still remains the same; the judge may prevaricate, but his prevarication, far from abolishing the law,

*Bullary of Benedict XIV, vol. 1, nos. 16, 30, 85.[3]
[3] Benedict XIV, *Bullarium;* forms vols. 15–17 of *Benedicti XIV . . . opera omnia . . . editio novissima,* 17 vols. (in typographia Bassanensi, sumptibus Remandini Veneti, 1767).

shows the strength of its dominion, since he can only escape it by a crime.*

The editors of *Denisart* declared in 1787: "We know of no Catholic church where divorce takes place, not excepting Poland." And after having concurred with the observations of the *Matrimonial Code,* they add: "A few years ago, Princess Saluskisambucko, whose marriage had been annulled in Poland, traveled to France. The prince of Nassau asked for her in marriage, and obtained her; the marriage was celebrated in Strasbourg." This marriage is thus not a proof of divorce, since it only took place because the first marriage had been annulled.†

A writer distinguished for his profound erudition, celebrated for his *True History of Mythical Times,*[6] M. l'abbé Guérin du Rocher, when consulted on the customs of Poland, where he had been a professor of canon law, replied, in writing and by word of mouth, "that the Council of Trent is accepted in Poland; that this church has no other doctrine on the indissolubility of marriage than that of Session 24 of the Council of Trent; that it professes its attachment to the Church and its perfect submission to the Holy See; that there are abuses in practice; that claims against marriages contracted several years previously are too easily accepted, on the basis of not having been free or of having been contracted with diriment impediments." Among the causes of these abuses, he indicts

---

Matrim. Code, new ed., 1770, vol. 1, p. 448.[4]
†*Collection of Recent Decisions,* vol. 6, word *Divorce,* p. 568.[5]
[4] Armand-Gaston Camus, *Code matrimonial, ou recueil complet des lois canoniques et civiles de France, des dispositions des conciles . . . sur les questions de mariage, nouvelle édition,* 2 vols. (Paris: Hérissant, 1770; orig. ed. 1766).
[5] Jean-Baptiste Denisart (1712–1765), *Collection de décisions nouvelles et de notions relatives à la jurisprudence,* 8th ed., various editors, 14 vols. (Paris: Veuve Desaint, 1783–1807). A standard work of French jurisprudence.
[6] Fr. Pierre-Marie-Stanislas Guérin du Rocher, *Histoire véritable des tems fabuleux,* 3 vols. (Paris: C.-P. Berton, 1776–1777).

the immense authority of the Polish lords, who, moving frequently from one estate to another, leave their places of residence uncertain.

A very eminent person, consulted on December 5, 1789 as to whether divorce occurs in Poland, replied, by a letter dated Warsaw, December 26, 1789, whose translation follows:

> The author of a new opuscule on divorce could assert nothing more untrue than that divorces are allowed in Poland as a custom tolerated by the Church. The grounds for annulment are treated in Poland as elsewhere, according to the disposition of the Council of Trent and the bull of Benedict XIV, *Dei miseratione*. Ever since the Catholic religion has been the dominant one, divorce or, more precisely, the notice of repudiation, has never been allowed among those who profess it. It cannot be denied that, whether by the incompetence of the judges, by a certain negligence in requiring and examining evidence in cases, or by the possibility of corrupting the judges and witnesses, there has been, and unfortunately still persists, a greater facility of annulling marriages there than elsewhere. As a result, the immortal Benedict XIV was obliged, in two forceful and energetic circular letters, to rebuke the Polish bishops for their scandalous indulgence in dissolving marriages. . . . Far from divorce being allowed there, the abuse (in dissolving them) derives from a certain facility of the bishops in accepting evidence for the nullity of marriage. . . . The nunciature certainly does its duty when a case of divorce is brought before it.

I have the Latin response, of January 15, 1790, to the superior of Saint Lazare, from the superior of the Warsaw seminary, consulted at my request. Here is an excerpt from it:

> In very promptly obeying your orders, I indicate here the sentiment of the Poles concerning divorce: never has there been any civil law in Poland allowing or approving divorce; never have I heard of any theologian who has distanced himself in his opinions from the evangelical doctrine, which the Council of Trent, principally, developed and declared in a more express manner; none of the consistories of the kingdom, as I have reason to know, think otherwise or follow any other rule in

practice. Collet's theology is taught in our seminaries, and in the four others which are under the guidance of the secular clergy. His sentiment on this point is very well known. . . . It is true that divorces occurred too often in Poland, principally at that time. As a result, Benedict XIV sent four briefs to our bishops, to pressure them, in the strongest manner, to combat this corruption. An anonymous English author, who has been translated into French, has dared to praise the Polish nation, as if, though professing the Catholic faith, it did not wish, as he asserts, to submit to the heavy yoke of the Roman pontiffs with regard to the indissolubility of marriage. Nevertheless, in all divorces the judicial forms are precisely observed. In consequence one party, in its own consistory, presents some diriment impediment to the other, by means of which it seeks juridically to prove the nullity of the marriage. The sentence is always appealed to the judgment of the metropolitan, and, if necessary, to the nuncio, or directly to Rome, in order to obtain two similar sentences, without which annulment is never declared. It is usual to allege two impediments in particular, namely, the lack of the presence of the parish priest, and the lack of consent, prevented by reverential fear. What furnishes a pretext for the first impediment is that, as the nobles and great men possess goods in various places, they object that the contractants had not lived long enough in the place where the marriage was contracted to have acquired legal residence there, or quasi-residence. In the second case, the parents sometimes swear and produce witnesses who swear that the party was constrained by force. These things having been alleged and proven, sentence is pronounced declaring the contract invalid. That these allegations are founded on truth is what is difficult to believe; nevertheless they customarily have their effect on the conscience; and hence, in our Poland, with regard to principles, the sentiment is the same as everywhere else, but the practice is sometimes not the same, because of the corruptions which have been introduced.

It is therefore a strange mistake in the *Methodical Encyclopedia*,[7] "Political Economy," vol. 2, part 1, word *Divorce*,

---

[7] *Encyclopédie méthodique*, 206 vols. (Paris: Pancouke, 1787–1825; various printings). The section on *Economie politique* comprises four volumes.

p. 121, to allege Poland as "a continuing example of a kingdom where divorce is included in the code of national laws and is practiced within the bounds of order." We are certain that no laws from this Code will be produced which authorize divorce properly speaking, and that it would be impossible to indicate a single case in which these laws authorize divorce.

It is therefore also erroneous to say, in the latest edition of the *Art of Verifying Dates,* chronology of the kings of Poland, vol. 2, p. 67, article *Micislas,* year 964, that the Poles have always considered divorce to be allowed. As this assertion, which is absent from the first two editions, is not supported by any evidence in the third, I had the editors asked to examine why it had been included. Here is D. Clément's reply: "What is said, in vol. 2, p. 67 of the *Art of Verifying Dates, on the basis of uncertain reports* concerning divorce which the Poles have always considered to be allowed, requires the testimony of witnesses, and needs to be clarified by persons well informed of the facts."

The testimony of the witnesses produced above has furnished the necessary clarification; all doubt must evaporate.

The author of *On Divorce*[8] has said (p. 2 of the introduction, and p. 55 of the work) that Poland accepts divorce. He has said, p. 57 of the work, "Poland, a Catholic kingdom, in which the Pope always has a legate (*he should have said a nuncio*), openly practices divorce." I asked him, during a visit with which he honored me, on what evidence he had asserted that divorce was allowed in Poland. He replied, with a candor which I take pleasure in doing justice to, that, "having received information concerning this point since the publication of the work, he had recognized that divorce is not allowed in Poland, but that marriages are often dissolved there, on the pretext of nullity."

---

[8] A reference to Albert Hennet's *Du divorce* (see note 1).

II.

Excerpt from the *Art of Verifying Dates,* vol. 3

Notice

With this third volume, we conclude a long and arduous effort, whose utility would be almost incalculable, if the execution corresponded to the importance of the subject. But the more we have advanced in this enterprise, the more imperfections we have discovered in it, as is shown by the additions and corrections we have placed at the end of each volume. Among the mistakes which have escaped us, the one which affects us the most is to have asserted, vol. 2, p. 73, following a number of modern authors, that the Poles have no scruples in allowing themselves divorce. It is true that, for several centuries, ecclesiastical discipline was extremely relaxed in Poland, etc.

After having exposed the abuse, Benedict XIV indicated its causes, etc.

From this M. de Rastignac very judiciously concludes that dissolutions of marriage in Poland are not based on the faculty of divorce, but on grounds for annulment, and on diriment impediments.

III.

Excerpt from the *Matrimonial Code,* vol. 1, p. 448

The author sets forth this objection: "Divorce takes place in Poland; the proof of this is that all marriages established through coercion are dissolved in that country; and as evidence of this coercion appears to be readily accepted, many people utter protests before marrying that they are only contracting by force." He replies: "The custom of Poland, far from establishing that divorce is authorized there, demonstrates the contrary," etc.

IV.

Consultation on Divorce, Requested in Poland in 1791

CONSULTATION

The purpose of this memoir is to make known the laws or customs followed on divorce, that is to say, on the act by which a legitimately contracted and consummated marriage is dissolved, with the capacity of the divorced spouses to establish a new marriage, each on his own account.

Is there a compendium or treatise of laws on divorce? In that case one would wish to see it.

For what causes is divorce granted?

REPLY

It is certain that it is very common in Poland to see two spouses leave each other, and establish new bonds afterwards.

This act is nevertheless not entirely a divorce, for it consists, not in dissolving a legitimate and valid marriage, but in declaring a marriage null and void.

It is nevertheless not entirely an annulment either; for what is null can produce no effect, and the children of a null marriage are illegitimate, whereas in Poland, this kind of nullity does not prevent the children from being legitimate.

There are no civil laws on divorce: in all matters of this kind, the regulations of the Church and the Papal bulls are precisely followed.

The reasons for which divorce can be requested are absolutely the same as those which nullify marriages in ecclesiastical law, which are known as *diriment im-*

pediments, included within five Latin lines, whose translation follows:

Error, condition, religious profession, holy orders, difference of religion, an existing first marriage, kinship, crime, honesty, impotence, violence.

Poland knows no other impediment particularly established, whether by synods or by any act of legislative power; but while, in the rest of the Catholic world, jurisprudence on the breaking of marriages has much restricted the above causes, in Poland it leaves them a great latitude, especially the last one, which is violence.

Is adultery a cause for divorce?

In Poland, adultery does not in any way dissolve marriage among Catholics.

Is incompatibility of temperament a cause for divorce?

No: in that event, spouses have recourse to one of the means of annulment, and most often their parents allow themselves to be accused of having forced them to marry.

Is the faculty of divorce equal for the husband and the wife?

As the contract of marriage is common to the husband and the wife, similarly the means of requesting divorce are common to them both.

How does the husband request divorce?

The request for divorce is made like other judicial requests, by setting forth, in the request or *libel,* the reasons one has to view the marriage as illegitimate and invalid, and by appearing in person to give evidence of this. Benedict XIV's bull of 1741, *Dei miseratione,* is observed.

Who are the first judges of divorce?

The same whom the canon law has established for all matters subject to ecclesiastical jurisdiction, that is, the bishops.

Who are the judges of appeal and of last resort?

One can regularly appeal from the bishop to the primate, from the primate to the Papal nuncio, and from the latter to the courts of Rome, or to the Pope directly, who ordinarily names judges delegated *ad hoc* in the second and third instance. Nevertheless, between the primate, the nuncio, and the courts of Rome, *predisposition* occurs, as in almost all cases subject to ecclesiastical jurisdiction.

What name, what title is born by a woman who is divorced and not remarried?

Polish divorce is, as has been said, an annulment which nevertheless differs in several points from real annulment: here, for example, in consideration of the good faith in which the divorced spouses lived together during the marriage, custom has established that, following divorce, the woman continues to bear the name of the husband she has left. There is no law concerning this; but she is recognized under that name before all courts and in all juridical acts.

ADDENDUM

SINCE the first edition of this work, divorce has been decreed; and one should doubtless refrain from resuming its discussion, if a law contrary to the nature of society were ever definitive, and if, until a contrary decision has been reached, the case did not remain pending before the court of reason.

When, in an enlightened nation, the legislator resolves to institute a bad or imperfect law, the motives of the administration must be carefully distinguished from the reasons for the law. The motives may be weighty, but the reasons are always false; and if policy does not allow the motives to be unveiled, prudence should forbid the reasons to be revealed.

Fortunately the legislator does not take the orator's discourse at his own risk, and it is possible to point out the errors of the latter, without failing in the respect owed to the former.

It must be admitted that, ever since writings began to appear for and against the indissolubility of the conjugal tie, weaker reasons have never been advanced in favor of divorce than those which preceded the decree authorizing it.

Those reasons have all been refuted in the course of this work; above all, the one which is insisted on with the greatest complaisance, "that the authorization of divorce is useless, dangerous, and out of place in a nascent people, whereas it is useful and necessary in an advanced one."

This assertion is belied by every page of history, where one sees polygamy or divorce tolerated by the laws of nascent peoples without danger to morals, as long as a sparse population, the habit of outdoor work, the mediocrity of fortunes, and the absence of the agreeable arts leave the passion of voluptuousness sleeping at the bottom of men's hearts, and allow the practice of divorce only as a resource against sterility, which is a misfortune among a nascent people alone; but this same faculty bears the most bitter fruit, and soon degenerates into a universal corruption, where the multiplication of men, the proximity of the sexes, the necessary inequality of ranks and riches, the taste for the arts, idleness and softness, awaken all the passions, summon all the pleasures, make marriage an attempt and divorce a game. We have before our eyes a striking example of this truth, even in advanced nations. Divorce is hardly practiced except among society's leisured classes, which are to the lower classes exactly what an advanced people is to a nascent one.

The assertion of the reporter is false in another and even more important sense: it supposes a Christian people to be a corrupted people, when a people can only be corrupted by the corruption of its laws, and not by the bad morals of a few individuals. When divorce, condemned by the religious laws of the greater number, is rejected by the morals of almost all, and examples of it are rare enough to be noticed, a people is good, and the legislator himself pays tribute to its goodness, both by the repugnance with which he proposes the faculty of dissolution and by the difficulties with which he surrounds its exercise. Would one not think, to listen to those who have written or spoken in favor of divorce, that France is a country of abomination, where marriage is a chain which all spouses are burning to break; and is it not singular that the same reason is given in France for authorizing divorce, of which still so few persons demand the faculty, which would be given in Turkey for not abolishing polygamy, which is of common right and generally practiced?

"Ah! doubtless," exclaims the reporter, "if one could, by some salutary law, suddenly purify the human species, the faculty of divorce would be unnecessary!" . . . ! Why make wishes when one can intimate orders? or rather, why chase chimeras of perfection when one has the most real and powerful means of order in one's hands? The human species can no

more be changed than any other, and man would not be what
he is, were he not as he is. The law is not made to purify the
species, but to repress penchants and direct them to good; and
what more can the legislator desire to repress and direct men's
penchants, and to impose strong and severe laws on them,
than to find a people long accustomed to their yoke, and
among which the morals of the greatest number are in harmony with the laws? An amazing thing! one could suddenly
subject a people to the law of military conscription, which
costs families so many tears, and yet one does not dare to
leave it under the law of indissolubility, which almost all families demand; as if it were easier to order an entire generation
of youth to hasten to the wars, than to force a few spouses to
remain united! Unfortunately one sees only the vices of a few,
and shuts one's eyes to the virtues of all: vice, which departs
from the rule, is more noticed than virtue, which remains
within the bounds of order; for the same reason that, on a
march, one only notices those who leave the ranks. Let us
dare to say, after a long and unhappy experience, that we must
make laws for the police in the cities, and laws for morals in
the countryside; and it is as inconsistent to take motives for
the laws from the capital, as to seek models for the arts in the
provinces.

SUMMATION
ON THE DIVORCE QUESTION

SUMMATION
ON THE DIVORCE QUESTION

> The statesman imitates nature, which, it appears, does not
> disturb the course of its operations to prevent the particular
> drawbacks arising from generally beneficial laws.

> Terrasson's *Philosophy*[1]

DIVORCE, requested in 1789 by a single *cahier,* the one presented by the Duke of Orléans, was decreed in 1792, around
the tragic days of September 2 and 3. It was a great case which
the nation lost, like so many others—and without being
heard—against those who claimed to represent it. Events have
given rise to an appeal before more enlightened judges; the
question has been resubmitted in happier circumstances, and
reason can appear to testify on its behalf. Already this good
cause has been pleaded in the legislative section of the Council
of State—eloquently so, in the opinion of more than a few; the
appeals court of Montpellier* has assumed the honor of its
defense; and the final remarks uttered here should only be
regarded like those summings up which, in major cases, the
contending parties present on the eve of the decision.

M. Maleville, the president of the Court of Cassation[2] and
one of the authors of the Civil Code, has accomplished this
important task in his writing *On Divorce and Separation.*[3] If

---

*It is noteworthy that the appeals courts of Montpellier and Nîmes, located
at the center of the departments with the most Protestants, have best
communicated the dangers of divorce. The appeals court of Riom has also
rejected it.

[1] The abbé Jean Terrasson, *La philosophie applicable à tous les objets de
l'esprit et de la raison* (Paris: Prault et fils, 1754).

[2] Roughly the French equivalent of the United States Supreme Court.

[3] Jacques, marquis de Maleville, *Du divorce et de la séparation de corps,* 50
pp. (Paris: Goujon fils, Year X [1801]). Maleville argues for the abolition of
divorce except for the cause of adultery.

one allows oneself to add a few observations to the wise, powerful, and luminous reasons he has presented against the faculty of divorce, they arise from the general manner in which the author of the present *Summation* has considered the questions relative to society, in a work too recent*[4] to be known to those who are called to pronounce on the divorce question. One will find in that work the development of the reasonings and facts which can only be indicated here.

One should not be surprised at the interest which a citizen, who though unknown is a sincere friend of his country, has taken in defending the indissolubility of the conjugal tie. He would like, if possible, to spare the government a major error and his country a major disaster.

Of Laws and Society

Society is the union of similar beings for the purpose of their reproduction and conservation.

Laws are the means which society uses to achieve its purpose, by repressing men's passions.

Laws are thus a good opposed to an evil, and an order established against disorder.

Society is domestic, political, and religious; it is family, State, and religion.

Laws, as the means of society, are therefore domestic, political, and religious.

Domestic society gathers men into family bodies; political society gathers men into State bodies; religious society, a

---

On Divorce, Considered in the Nineteenth Century.
[4] Bonald is not engaging in false modesty here. *On Divorce* was probably published in the second half of 1801 and the Summation in the fall of that year. The Council of State began its discussion of the proposed Civil Code on 4 Thermidor, Year IX (July 23, 1801)—right around the time of publication of *On Divorce*.

universal bond, *a religare,*[5] gathers, or should gather men, families, and States into one body.

The law of marriage is a domestic law; the law of succession to the throne is a political law; the law of established religion is a religious law.

All these laws are *natural,* but of a different nature; for the family is natural to man; the political state is natural to families; and religion is natural to men, families, and States.

Of Marriage

Marriage is a law directed against man's inconstancy, a means to repress the intemperance of his desires.

The end of marriage is not the pleasures of man, since he tastes them outside of marriage.

The end of marriage is not only the reproduction of man, since this reproduction can also take place without marriage.

But the end of marriage is the reproduction and, above all, the conservation of man, since this conservation cannot, in general, take place outside of marriage, or without marriage.

The effect of marriage is therefore the perpetuation of humankind; for humankind consists, not of the children who are produced, but of the men who are conserved.

Therefore marriage is a good law; for everything which conserves beings is well or good.

The family, composed of the father, mother, and children, is an *actual* society made up of three persons: power, agent or minister, and subject, like every society.

The marriage which precedes the family and produces it, made up of the man and the woman, is a *potential* society.

Nature has not fixed the term of this *potential,* or the arrival of children.

[5] "From 'to bind.' "

Thus, the non-arrival of children is not a *reason* to dissolve marriage, because they could still arrive (for if there were *impotence,* there would have been no marriage), still less to contract a new one, whose fertility is equally speculative. Once children arrive, the society, from being *potential,* becomes *actual;* if children have been produced, there are men to conserve or educate, and there is a *reason* not to dissolve the marriage; for one must talk *reason* to legislators.

If marriage is a potential society, and if this society is made up of three persons, the father, mother, and child, then marriage is truly a contract between three persons, two of whom are present, one of whom (the child) is absent, but is represented by public power, guarantor of the commitment made by the two spouses to form a society; for public power always represents the absent person in the family: the child before its birth, the father after his death.* The contract formed between three persons cannot be broken by two, to the prejudice of the third, the weakest one in the society; and this third person can never consent to a rupture which is wholly to his prejudice, because he is always a minor in the family, even when he has reached his majority in the State.

Marriage is a natural society, not a commercial association. The stakes are unequal, since the man contributes protection and strength, the woman, the needs of weakness: the results, in the event of separation, are unequal as well, since the man leaves with all his authority, while the woman does not leave with all her dignity, and since, out of everything she brought into the marriage—virginal purity, youth, beauty, fertility, reputation, wealth—she can only, in the event of dissolution, recover her money.

Marriage is therefore naturally indissoluble.

The ancients thought so; consider Virgil:

---

*See the development of this reason in *On Divorce, Considered in the Nineteenth Century.*

Connubio jungam stabili, propriamque dicabo.[6]

Consider Tacitus, in his work on the Germans: "Happier and wiser are those cities where only virgins are allowed to marry, and open their hearts only once to the desires and hopes of a wife; they receive a husband as one receives a body and a soul," etc.

Consider Dionysius of Halicarnassus: "The more ancient laws of Rome, which prohibited divorces, are extremely praised by him," says M. Maleville. "Wonderful was the harmony, says the historian, which this inseparable union of interests produced between married persons."[7]

The natural indissolubility of the conjugal tie was recognized, prior to 1792, by all modern authorities, even those that permitted its dissolution. The authors of the proposed Civil Code proclaim this natural indissolubility in explicit terms; the reporter for the Court of Cassation, at the very time he was asking for the dissolution of the conjugal tie, went so far as to say: "Marriage is a perpetual society in its wish." And what are the wishes of perfection which man, assisted by the laws, is unable to accomplish?

Of Separation and Divorce

If the union of the spouses is a natural bond, their separation can become a necessary misfortune.

The separation of goods and bodies (which is called *a mensa et a toro*) without dissolution of the bond remedies all the disorders of the disunion of hearts: reason is satisfied with

---

[6] "I shall join her to you in a lasting marriage and pronounce her your own." Virgil, *Aeneid* 1.73 = 4.126.

[7] The quotation is actually from David Hume's essay *Of Polygamy and Divorces,* and is accurately identified as such by Maleville, op. cit., p. 15.

it; but the passions go further, and demand the dissolution of marriage and the capacity to form new bonds: this is what is called *divorce*.

The first care of legislators is to prescribe, to facilitate the execution of the laws; and the first care of legislators with regard to the law on divorce is to prohibit it, in some sense, and if possible to render its execution impossible.

Will the partisans of divorce say that it is a disorder opposed to a still greater disorder? What greater disorder is there in society than the very dissolution of society?

Will they say that divorce is a cure rather than a law? It is marriage which is a cure for the inconstancy of our desires; and divorce, which breaks marriage, destroys the cure, delivers man to his inconstancy, and is consequently an evil.

But before examining the arguments presented for the faculty of divorce, and the facts alleged in its favor, it is necessary to examine the two contrasting opinions held by its partisans.

Of Free Divorce and Legal Divorce

Nothing more clearly shows the viciousness of the principle of divorce than to witness those who accept it seeking a cure for the cure itself, by placing restrictions on it which reason cannot approve, or by making it depend on impossible conditions.

There are, in effect, two opinions on divorce. Some would like divorce to be as free, as easy, as marriage itself. They would demand no legal, proven cause for divorce to be pronounced. Others wish to limit divorce to certain cases specified in advance, and subject to legal proof at the time of the event.

These opinions have been argued before the Court of Cassation, and it is clear that their partisans have been unable to reconcile them, since they were presented in two opposing reports.

The system of free divorce, it must be admitted, is more consistent than the system of legal divorce; and on this basis alone, it is either all good or all bad; for consistency in reasoning is a certain proof that there is entire truth or entire error in the thought. It is an equation which gives an equally correct result whether it gives a positive or negative quantity. "If divorce is an evil," say the defenders of the first system, "it should be rejected; if it is a cure, why postpone it or make it so difficult to obtain? But here only the sick man knows his sickness and can judge the need for the cure. The offenses which trouble domestic harmony and make divorce necessary are purely domestic, and can only be known, felt, and judged by domestic persons; just as the crimes which disturb the public peace can only be known and judged by public persons. The civil magistrate is obliged to unite the spouses upon the notice they give him of their wish to unite; why, to disunite them, should he require anything other than the information they give him of their wish to leave each other?" That is what the reporter for free divorce demonstrates most clearly. "To reduce the admissible reasons for divorce to specific causes," he says, "is to do nothing in most cases. It is to propose a cure for misery on condition that it shall be unable to cure those forms of misery which are most common, most hurtful, and most unbearable. . . . For where in a case of divorce is a fact which a husband or wife can present in evidence? Where is one which they can prove? Where is one which can be judged?" (*See the opinion of the Court of Cassation.*)

These arguments are embarrassing; the partisans of legal divorce cannot reply to them without attacking the principle itself; and indeed, the intervention of public authority in domestic disputes is as out of place as the intervention of the people in public judgments can be dangerous.

But however consistent this theory may be, it is unworkable in practice; and it is this which demonstrates its falsity. Thus, after having with great effort established the need for free divorce in a lengthy discourse, the reporter concludes by proposing numerous limitations on it; and it is truly curious to see the efforts he makes to discover a means to reconcile the chimera of an ideal freedom with the possibility of a practical execution.

"He allows divorce only after five years of marriage and before twenty years.

"He requires that the husband be at least thirty years old and at most fifty; and that the wife be at least twenty-five years old and at most forty-five.

"He wants the person who instigates the divorce to be forbidden to remarry for two years after the divorce is pronounced.

"Finally (and this is the most inscrutable restriction), he wants to forbid that a person divorce twice *in the same manner* in the course of his life"; as if the laws could prevent a man whom they allow to marry more than one woman from being unhappy more than once!

One can see the reason for setting the age of majority at twenty-one to twenty-five years of age, because it is natural for the mind to have acquired its full strength when the organs destined to serve it have reached their full growth. One can also see the reason for the law which limits the requirement that fathers consent to their children's marriages to twenty-five years of age for girls and thirty for boys, because this is already the age of wisdom, and, further advanced, it would no longer be the age of marriage. After all, children only suffer from failing to obey, and the law was obliged to limit the age of disobedience to the age of youth. But where is the reason which requires that divorce, although necessary and permitted at a certain period in marriage and a certain time in life, is no longer permitted a month earlier or a month later, even if it is equally necessary? Why forbid the cure when you cannot prevent the disorder? Why so much liberty at one time and so little liberty at another? Why, when a divorce is adjudged, should the party which wishes to form new bonds be subjected to a two-year novitiate, after the law has allowed it to break a twenty-year marriage? As if these problems were not great enough, the reporter for free divorce *wishes it to be sold to the spouses at the price of that which they hold most dear.* Is it justice which will sell divorce? Is it the guilty party which will pay its price? And if it should be both of them: Will it be in favor of the children? And if there are no children? Will it be the instigator who pays the price of the sale? But if it is a virtuous woman who has already endured a husband's ill-usage, will divorce be for her like trial by fire, in which the accused was forced to burn his hands in order to clear himself of the crime of theft? When one sees the reporter trying to repair the immense disorders of his system with his little laws, one thinks of workers multiplying the props around a crumbling building, or a carpenter busy closing the leaks which spring open all over a sinking ship. Hence the authors of the Civil Code have taken the side of legal divorce, as has the second reporter for the Court of Cassation. They have even specified five grounds for divorce. The Council of State, if it admits the faculty of divorce, *quod dii avertant,*[8] will decide in favor of legal divorce, on the basis of specific grounds, of which only the last two, murder and adultery, are worthy of consideration.

Of the Accusation of Murder

Here inextricable difficulties arise. Is there only an intent to murder? —There is not even a basis for accusation. Is there

---

[8] "Which may the gods avert."

an act and an attempt to murder? —There are grounds for capital punishment; for one would surely not wish to forbid prosecutors the duty to pursue the party guilty of such a heinous crime, or to grant spouses a privilege of homicide. Will the death penalty be abolished specifically for conjugicide? —It must be abolished for all crimes. Will the sentence be commuted? —What would be the motive? All the penalty or no penalty; and reason, in this case, knows no middle ground between the scaffold and a second marriage. But what would actually happen if the prosecutor were allowed to pursue the murdering spouse? In France, where a delicate sentiment of generosity and even of humanity prohibited a master from denouncing a faithless servant, a still better-founded sentiment would never allow a spouse to deliver the friend of his youth and the mother of his children to the executioner. He could not separate himself from her without divorcing her, nor divorce her without compromising her life; he will prefer to allow her to remain beside him, if he cannot distance himself from her; he will fear for his family the unhappy distinction of appearing in *causes célèbres,* and he will not want to brand his children with the mark of ignominy.

The crime of a mother is a heavy burden.

And, I dare say, the French spirit—that vigorous principle of such decent morals, such generous practices, such glorious actions—would be totally extinguished if we could become accustomed to seeing spouses tear each other from the marriage bed to drag each other to the scaffold. And, too, how is one to prove a domestic homicide—this treason prefaced by a kiss, this poison offered in the marriage cup, this fatal noose tightened in the shadows by fraternal hands; this murder, finally, to which in this unhappy age it would be so easy to lend the color of suicide? The Roman laws did not admit parricide;

our own would forestall a still more heinous crime; for what human affections can equal the *friendship of nature,* in the expression of M. Bernardin de Saint-Pierre, and the ineffable union of man and wife?

Of Adultery

The proposed Civil Code distinguishes the adultery of the husband from the adultery of the wife, and reason acknowledges this distinction. The multiplicity of women can conduce to the goal of nature; the multiplicity of men distances itself from it. The adultery of the wife destroys the family, the adultery of the husband afflicts only the heart of the wife.

The adultery of the husband only provides grounds for divorce insofar as the husband houses the concubine under the same roof as the wife; and in this provision, the proposed law considers less the adultery in itself than the outrage committed against the wife. But what a vast field does such a provision not open to license and bad morals? Would a husband given over to outside affections merely have to place their object beside him and in his house, in order to rid himself of his wife and marry his concubine at one stroke? This law, oppressive in the highest degree, punishes the wife for her own misfortunes, and crowns the husband's disorders with full success. And what audacious rival could not persuade her fascinated lover to introduce her into his house, sure, by this means, legally to replace the legitimate wife?

And, in another regard, how serious an assault is it on the husband's authority, and consequently on domestic peace and good morals, to offer a violent and jealous woman such a means to interpret the affections of her spouse toward all the women who may live under the same roof; to torment him with endless suspicions and continual threats of accusation; to drag him, perhaps, before the courts in order to dispute his actions, divulge his disorders, or defame his virtues?

Adultery on the part of the wife must be proved either by a public scandal or by writings in her hand. But in the first case, there can be no public scandal when usage allows a woman to go by day or by night, alone or in a group, to lunch as to a ball, with any man, provided he is not her own. As to proof by writing—the only external evidence which the law recognizes—it is supremely dangerous to make the evidence for a capital crime depend on certain intrinsic conditions to the exclusion of all others.

If the law admitted evidence of murder only to the extent that witnesses had seen it committed in broad daylight, it would suffice, to escape the law, not to commit it before or after a certain hour. There are laws in England which are so specific, with regard to the circumstances of a crime, that it is possible to incur a severe penalty for beating a man, but to have no legal liability for killing him. In this instance, adulterous lovers will correspond without writing, as they hear each other without speaking. Then the best thing a father will be able to do for his daughter's happiness will be to give her no notion of this unhappy art; for, thanks to modern chemistry and its discoveries in the art of removing handwriting, a letter which a woman has written, even to her husband in the intimacy of marriage, could, through circumstances which are easy to create and a signature which is easy to change, become, in treacherous hands, the means of her ruin, the text and proof of an accusation of adultery.

And let it not be said that I suppose men to be more wicked than they are; for to refute such an accusation, it suffices to cite the first report of the Court of Cassation. To hear the reporter tell it, France is Tartarus, and she is only inhabited by demons. The number of unhappy spouses and of marriages which present the spectacle of *victims attached to their tor-*

turers is *incalculable;* for it is extremely remarkable that the same doctrines which deny man's native or original corruption invariably exaggerate the extent of his social corruption. For my part, I am very far from thinking that morals in France are as depraved as the reporter is pleased to imagine. There are unhealthy spirits who, to judge things soundly, would require a change of air. They see only Paris, and should consider the distant departments, where a divorce today would still be a real phenomenon. But it is certain that disorder is advancing step by step; that, through the faculty of divorce, morals in France will fall into an extreme corruption; and that the reporter, in thinking he was describing what is, has only proclaimed what will be.

Finally, when two spouses, mutually accusing each another of murder and adultery, fail to prove their cases, the judges will send them back home *in peace;* and the intervention of public authority, having failed to protect either the woman's life or the man's honor, will have had no effect but to entertain the public with scandals and slanders, to divide families, and to render a wife notorious or a husband ridiculous.

All these limitations on the faculty of divorce, all the obstacles raised against it, may make divorce difficult to obtain, but only indissolubility makes marriage honorable. And what does it matter if divorces are rare, if spouses can never be indissolubly united? It is not difficulties which must be opposed to man's desires, for difficulties only inflame them, but the impossibility of satisfying them altogether. In the course of his passions, man stops only at the barrier which halts the Almighty himself: before the impossible.

Everything which is irritating in an indissoluble marriage becomes unbearable in a marriage subject to dissolution. Spouses then are like miserable captives who have partly opened the door of their prison and are constantly engaged in widening the gap to make a way out. In an indissoluble marriage, the woman is *of* the man; in a dissoluble marriage, the woman is *to* the man;* and the man, strong when she is weak, young when she is young no longer, has as many means as desires to dismiss her. These are laws for slaves, not laws for children; laws of fear, not laws of love; and it is better to tolerate adultery and even murder than to destroy society in order to punish them.

Reasons Alleged in Favor of Divorce

Objections must be answered.

Can one condemn divorced spouses to the loneliness of celibacy? But should one reward weakness or crime by allowing a second marriage? They will live in concubinage. The law of divorce only remedies this problem through adultery, for the pronouncement of municipal authority legalizes the tie and does not legitimize it.

The abuses of divorce will be minimized by reducing them to specific causes. This would only present the passions with infallible means to satisfy themselves, and the *specific* causes are signposts on a road.

Marriages increase population. Population only grows through families; and there is no family today if it can end tomorrow.

How can we leave together spouses who hate each other? Why separate brothers who love each other, and who, raised by hostile hands, will hate each other one day?

The law does not require divorce. In the times in which we live, to allow divorce is to require prostitution.

Not only should the law prohibit divorce; it should proclaim

*In the Christian religion, the woman is *of* the man, *bone of his bone, flesh of his flesh, and they are two in one flesh;* among the pagans, the woman was *to* the man, and he could assign her possession, like that of a piece of furniture, by year of enjoyment.

the indissolubility of marriage. Divorce is an oppression of woman, even when she herself provokes it; for in the eyes of reason, an unhappy woman is always less to be pitied than a divorced one.

Will it be said: *Divorce presents no drawbacks among simple peoples?* It is because they make no use of it. The rarity of divorce is the effect of the simplicity of morals, as the rarity of illness is a sign of good health. It is not its cause; and to believe that one can return an advanced people to simple morals, with complaisances which are only appropriate to a nascent people, is to attempt to return a grown man to the condition of infancy by putting him in a cradle.

Our morals are corrupted. Purify morals, and do not corrupt the laws.

Our morals oppose the law of indissolubility. Reason has never more clearly recognized the need for it. These Romans and these Greeks, whose virtues and morals are constantly vaunted to us, applauded plays in which the rape of slaves, traffic in women, and prostitution were the ordinary elements of drama; while the French, of whose corruption we hear so much, reject even the appearance of divorce in their theaters. They take offense at an indecent word, and are disgusted by the licentiousness of the English theater. The simplicity of our forefathers honored the bastard almost as much as the legitimate son; and we, in our degeneracy, mark with infamy the offspring of a union unrecognized by the law. We only hear of the corruption of morals, which has been tolerated and increased by governments more concerned with things than with people; but nothing is heard of the progress of reason, enlightened by Christianity, of this public reason which has brought us back from so far to the principles of order, and which brings us back without effort or violence, because order is what is most in conformity with our reason and the natural law of the universe. Let weak men say what they like; never, for the promulgation of *severe* laws, has the government had greater support from the strength of our reason, or greater motives from the weakness of our morals.

Finally, and this is the most specious objection: *The indissolubility of the conjugal tie is a religious law, and the civil law of France recognizes no religion.* The law of indissoluble marriage is a domestic law, as the law of abstinence is a religious law. If one views it as religious because it is consecrated by religion, why not also view as religious, why recognize as civil, the prohibition of robbery and murder, which religion also consecrates, and indeed, consecrates even more expressly and clearly than the prohibition of divorce? The reason is that the Christian religion has made dogmas of all that nature had made principles, and that marriage, as all parties agree, is naturally indissoluble. England herself, whether or not she views marriage as a religious law, gives Parliament the sole power to dissolve it. *But one sect, in France, calls for divorce.* That is a mistake, it is only a party; and the Protestants themselves have long since recognized its abuse, as witness Mme. Necker, David Hume, and the English Parliament; as witness their morals in France, which, in agreement with the laws, rejected divorce.

Moreover, let us dare to return to principle: governments are instituted to make men better and the family stronger.

The law of the indissolubility of the conjugal tie is a perfect law; its opponents themselves acknowledge this, since they only criticize it for its perfection; it is not impracticable, since it is practiced everywhere. The government therefore does not wrong—what am I saying?—it benefits those whom it raises to a more perfect state, and it oppresses only those whom it reduces to a less perfect one. And do not object on the ground of religious belief, for divorce is an action, not a belief; and, even on questions of dogma, the reformed religion has placed itself under the authority of civil government, and it is this which constitutes its error and the real weakness of States which seek a support in it.

Facts Alleged in Favor of Divorce

It is necessary, before entering into the discussion of the facts alleged in favor of divorce, to pause over an assertion by one of the reporters for the Court of Cassation, M. Target; an assertion contradicted by reason and history alike, but which has achieved a certain currency among those who consult neither.

"Some," says this reporter, "must have told themselves that divorce was not good for civil society, and that it had already been tried. I believe this is an error. No, divorce of the first moments is not *habitual* divorce in a peaceful State; no, divorce applied to marriages contracted under the *iron rule* of indissolubility is not divorce applied to those contracted under the rule of a law which is *gentler and more compatible with human nature.*" And earlier on he says: "It should be noted that the greatest abuse, not only of bad laws, but also of good ones, erupts at the time of their birth."

In the first place, the vices of a law must be distinguished from the abuses man adds to it. A good law has no vices; but it is subject to men's passions in the course of its execution. A bad law is bad both as a result of man's abuses and as a result of its own vices. In a word, divorce is a weak or bad law, even when it is not used; indissolubility is a good law, even when it is abused.

If divorce became *habitual* in a nation, the non-dissolution of marriage would be the *accidental* state. Divorce would therefore be the general law and marriage the exception. If divorce became *habitual,* the State would be peaceful; yes, with the calm of death. It would have passed from frenzy to lethargy. *Divorce of the first moments is not habitual divorce in a peaceful State:* Does the reporter mean to say that divorce will become less frequent in proportion as it becomes more habitual, or that it will become less scandalous in proportion as it becomes more frequent? Does he mean to say that the law of divorce will fall into desuetude, like some ancient decree fixing the hours of a market, the place of a fair, or the name of a village? Let us search history for proof of this assertion, as contrary to the principles of reason as to the facts of society: *Divorce of the first moments is not habitual divorce in a peaceful State.*

The form of divorce allowed among the Jews was not the same as ours. The repudiation which their law accorded to the husband alone *was an act of jurisdiction, even when it was not an act of justice;* whereas divorce, allowed among the Greeks and ourselves to the wife against the husband, *is an act of rebellion, even when it is excused by its motives.* I know very well that the philosophical doctrines seek to establish equality between husband and wife; but when it comes to practice, one encounters nature, which opposes its eternal order to the transient disorder of human theories, and forces the legislator to acknowledge, to declare that the woman is subordinate in the family as in the State; and that, even in domestic society, she *has* authority only to the extent that she is *authorized* by he who *is* authority.

In the early days of Rome, repudiation was allowed to the husband alone. Similarly, it was allowed to the husband alone in the early days of Greece. It is noteworthy that the laws of all ancient peoples, as one goes back in time, increasingly resemble the laws of the Jews (and one even finds some examples of Judaic repudiation in the early days of our own history), just as the laws of modern peoples increasingly resemble the laws of Christianity as modern peoples advance in their social career.

Be that as it may, among the Jews, Romans, and Greeks, *divorce of the first moments was not habitual divorce in a peaceful State;* for divorce among the Jews, which was so rare in *the first moments* that one scarcely finds a single case of it in their history, became so *habitual* toward the end of the republic and *in a peaceful State* that their most learned doctors taught that a husband could dismiss his wife to marry one more beautiful, or merely because she had burned the soup. Among the Romans, divorce, which was so rare in *the first moments* that five centuries elapsed without a single case of it, became so *habitual* in later years that, according to Seneca, women counted their years by the number of their husbands rather than the names of the consuls; and the emperor Augustus (a unique case in history!) had to pass laws requiring the citizens to marry.

Among the Greeks, as among all peoples, divorce must have been rare in *the first moments;* but in the *peaceful state,* the *habitual* contempt for women and the degeneration of all natural laws were carried to a level of excess which a phrase of Plutarch's, from his *Moral Works,* suffices to convey: "As to true love, it is well known that women have no part in it." M. de Montesquieu says that Plutarch speaks like his century. What a way to speak and what a century!

Among all peoples, *the greatest abuse of the law did not erupt at the time of its birth;* for all peoples began by allowing repudiation to the husband alone, and all ended by allowing the wife to dismiss the husband. The legislators who introduced this *gentle* law were Herod, Domitian, and Solon. One was a harsh law, the other was a bad law and a law against nature; and woman was exposed both to her husband's inconstancy and to her own.

Among those modern nations which allow the dissolution of the conjugal tie, divorce, more scandalous in *the first moments* because of its novelty, has not become less abusive by becoming more *habitual.* Divorce was common in Geneva, in Switzerland, in Berlin, in the *peaceful state* of the Protestant nations; for it is positively false that the dissolution of marriage is allowed in Poland. In England, where divorce is pronounced only for the cause of adultery, where the guilty party is forbidden to remarry, where the dissolution must be pronounced by Parliament, where, finally, according to *Blackstone,* vol. 2, ch. 7, divorce is only an exception to the general law of indissolubility; in England, divorce today so little resembles divorce in *the first moments,* and in becoming *habitual* has become so troublesome and abusive, that, says M. Maleville:

> Although the costs of such an act and such proceedings are enormous, nevertheless the abundance of gold and the corruption of morals made adultery and divorce so common that, in 1779, they aroused the concern of Parliament, and suggestions were put forward, notably that of the Duke of Richmond, to abolish divorce outright. Parliament, however, limited itself to placing new restrictions on it; adulterous men and women were forbidden to remarry for a year; but experience has shown this remedy to be unsuccessful, and recently complaints have arisen again on this subject in Parliament.

Finally we ourselves, since we have been *in a peaceful state,* have discovered that divorce is becoming *habitual,* and this is precisely what is causing alarm among virtuous men and arousing the concern of the government. Divorce, it is true, caused more of a stir in *the first moments;* but it has not become less frequent since then by being less noticed, and *its greatest abuses did not erupt at the time of its birth.* As common today in Paris as it was at the time of its origin, it has begun to reach the provinces, and from the towns it is spreading to the countryside. There were, according to M. Maleville, even more divorces in the last eleven months of Year IX of the revolution than in the whole of Year VIII; and divorce has become so *habitual,* following the wish of the reporter, that it can be calculated that, of every five marriages in Paris, one will *habitually* be broken.

It is equally false that "divorce applied to marriages contracted under the *iron rule* of indissolubility is not divorce applied to those contracted under the rule of a law which is *gentler and more compatible with human nature.*" For—other than the fact that it is a cruel mockery to describe the law of divorce as *gentle and compatible with human nature,* when it carries to the highest pitch the tyranny of the husband and the oppression of the woman and child—divorce, which in *the first moments* could only attack marriages contracted under the previous law, today no longer attacks those contracted under this *iron* law, but those contracted under the *gentle* law of 1792, and sometimes even marriages contracted eight days ago. One does not speak of the authorities cited in favor of divorce—*Montesquieu, Grotius, Milton,* the English, German, and Genevan publicists, etc., etc. After the experience of the revolution, which destroyed reputations of more than one kind, France has, if I may be allowed this expression, completed her studies in philosophy. Having finished her courses, she can evaluate her teachers; and she must, on political matters, consult her reason, enlightened today by facts far better than it was by books.

General Observations on Divorce

1. The English Parliament wished to abolish divorce, and it will abolish it; for, when once a nation has felt the viciousness of a law, it cannot rest until it has been changed. There are a number of peoples in Europe which, having left the perfect state of the natural laws of society some centuries ago, and having fallen into corruption since that time, are saying like the Prodigal Son: "I shall go back where I began."*

It would be dishonorable for France to descend to an imperfect state which her rival would be the first to leave, and we are not in the habit of receiving such examples.

2. The oppression the government would impose on the

---

*The English Parliament deliberated on the abolition of black slavery and the abolition of divorce at the same time. We hastened, for our misfortune, to forestall, on the first question, a decree which it did not wish to render, and which was only proposed to tempt us, and we decreed divorce, which was neither in our morals nor our laws.

thirty-nine fortieths of the nation which regard divorce as a crime would be the most severe the nation has suffered in a decade, since it would be a moral oppression and the corruption of morality by the laws. The government, for the defense of the State, has the power to destroy the family; but under no circumstances whatever can it have the right to corrupt it.

And not only would it corrupt the family by the license it would give man's desires, but it would banish happiness and peace from it as well, by the hatreds which divorce would not fail to incite between families. What deep resentments would not be provoked among this sensitive people, precise appraiser of favors and insults; what tears, what blood would not flow from the affront to a girl, often innocent, sent back without honor and without a name to the home and parents that she, happy and proud of the beauty of a maiden and the dignity of a wife, had left a short time before! And if the Frenchman should degenerate to the point of becoming insensitive to such an affront, he would doubtless soon fall into the same excess of degradation as a neighboring people which, even in the most opulent circumstances, evaluates the weakness of a woman, the crime of a seducer, and the shame of a husband in pounds, shillings, and pence, and sues for the total on expert estimates.

3. A small part of the nation views divorce as tolerated, and did not even make use of this toleration; all the rest views it as a crime, and if there are a few who view it as a good, it is not for them that laws are made. To allow divorce to all would be gratuitously to perpetuate religious disagreements, fertile source of political dissension; to forbid it to all, as was proposed for England in its Parliament, would be to fulfill a duty toward the greater part of the nation without inflicting any wrong on the other part; it would be above all to prepare a path for religious unity, which is the first object of any wise government, but which it should never expect from anything but education and time.

For the opinion that the religious must be carefully separated from the civil has not yet attained prescriptive status in society, though disseminated under a thousand forms for the last century. Government should doubtless not command everything which religion prescribes to man as personal; but it should allow nothing which religion forbids as fundamental in society, still less should it forbid anything which religion commands. Indeed, sometimes government may precede religion, and forbid what religion tolerated only for a time. Religion directs will; the civil laws repress actions. To separate the direction of wills and the repression of actions in society is to separate the soul from the body in man; it is to materialize society, to annihilate it, by destroying the principle of its strength and progress. The indestructible strength, the incontestable preeminence of France, consisted in this harmony of the religious and the civil, more perfect in France, perhaps, than in any other nation, and which, by giving her constitution that theocratic element which distinguished it, made the *Very Christian* State the very powerful State.

4. Some, who deplore the weakness of our penchants better than they judge the progress of our reason, would like to restore us to better morals through a wisely restrained divorce. They wish to create good morals in order to create good laws; they cite the ancients at every pretext, and this celebrated adage of one of their poets: *Quid leges sine moribus vanae proficiunt?*[9] Ancient times bear no resemblance to modern times. Morals were visible among the ancients, that is to say the observation of domestic laws rather than political ones; and this must be so, because the ancients, located nearer the beginning, were closer to the time when the family preceded the State. Their political laws, when they had any, were ex-

[9] "What avail vain laws without morals?" Horace, *Odes* 3.24.35–36. This quotation serves as an epigraph to the abbé Gabriel Bonnot de Mably's *Entretiens de Phocion* (Amsterdam, 1763). Bonald attacks Mably along with Rousseau in the *Essai analytique* ("Analytical Essay"; Paris: Le Clère, 1800).

tremely imperfect. M. de Montesquieu goes so far as to say that the ancients even lacked the idea of a government established on fundamental laws. In this state of things, morals, far from finding a support in the political and religious laws, found in them only inconsistency, absurdity, license, and disorder. And, for instance, what humanity was not required in morals, in places where the State and even religion presented the people with the spectacle of homicide as an entertainment, or as a sacrifice acceptable to the gods? What temperance was not required in places where prostitution was part of public worship; in places where the most unrestricted divorce was allowed and abominable loves authorized? Certainly, such laws could only expect their corrective from morals, which nevertheless resisted only a short time among the Romans, and even less among the Greeks, under the powerful influence of these corrupting laws. But since *the highest wisdom has made itself heard* to men, as Jean-Jacques Rousseau says, and the knowledge of the natural relationships of man with his fellows has served as the basis for the law codes of societies, reason has become public, the laws have attained perfection, and so morals, far from operating as a corrective to weak, disordered, and variable laws, have found their rule in strong and immutable ones; so that it became possible to reverse the maxim of the ancients and say, *Quid mores sine legibus,* etc.;[10] and it was no longer necessary to await the restoration of morals from sources other than the goodness of the laws. Thus it would be senseless to think that men's passions, aroused by the license of the arts, will be more moderate when they have greater means to satisfy themselves, or that after fifty years of divorce it will be easier to return to indissolubility.

5. I shall conclude with a thought worthy to hold the attention of statesmen:

The nations which allow divorce or polygamy are the weakest of all European nations, less because they lack strength for

10 "What [avail] morals without laws?"

aggression than because they lack strength for stability and conservation. France, which rejects divorce, was the strongest of Christian nations, because she was the most reasonable, the most natural in her laws. If she decrees the dissolubility of the conjugal tie, with a few restrictions even as she allows its dissolution, she will solemnly proclaim—in the nineteenth century, after three centuries of inquiry, knowledge, and enlightenment, in the face of the universe and in the presence of all the great minds she has produced, those of Descartes, Bossuet, Fénelon, Domat, and d'Aguesseau—she will proclaim as a principle, THAT THE LAWS MUST BE WEAKER TO THE EXTENT THAT MORALS ARE MORE CORRUPT; and that when men no longer see anything in marriage but an enjoyment and make a game of license, then divorce must be the penalty for adultery; change, the cure for inconstancy; pleasure, the restraint on voluptuousness. Divorce was allowed three centuries ago because men thought they had discovered a toleration of it in the divine oracles; today, it will be decreed exclusively as a concession to human passions. This law which was proclaimed in 1792 as a necessary *consequence* of a system of destruction, to the cries of the slaughtered victims, will be presented ten years later as a basis, a *principle,* in a system of rebuilding, amidst songs of triumph and peace. At the very time that the English, tired of its license, are proclaiming the noble intention to cast off its yoke, the French will receive it, and in a still more licentious form; the shameful weakness of their laws will avenge the peoples vanquished by their arms, and, like the Romans,

Luxuria incubuit, victumque ulciscitur orbem.[11]

But if a single false idea can deprave a man, what, for a nation, would be the effect of an absurd principle which it

---

[11] "Luxury has settled on us and avenges our conquest of the world." Juvenal 6.293.

makes the basis for its legislation? Public reason, of which France was the voice in Europe, would be obscured by it; the common legislation of Christian nations would be shaken; and it would be demonstrated to man, who sees in the superiority of enlightenment the only title to preeminence among civilized peoples, that France has fallen below her prerogative, and that the scepter of Europe is going to pass to other hands.

INDEX

INDEX

to On Divorce

adultery
  as a ground for divorce, 90,
    112, 137, 138, 164, 183–
    186, 191–192
Aguesseau, Henri-François d',
  197
Akiba (rabbi), 82
Ambrose, Saint, 154
Amphilocus, 113n
Aristides, 9, 96
aristocracy, 61, 88, 89
Aristotle, 17
Augustine, Saint, 24, 98, 154
Augustus, 191
Aulus Gellius, 90

Basil, Saint, 113n
Benedict XIV, 155–156, 158–
  159, 161, 165
Bergier, the abbé Nicolas-
  Sylvestre, 80
Beza, Theodore, 117
Blair, Hugh, 125
Bossuet, Jacques-Bénigne,
  bishop of Meaux, 32, 58, 197
Bucer, Martin, 137

Cagliostro, Alessandro, 51n
Calvin, John, 101, 103, 137, 139
Carvilius Ruga, 89, 90
Cato the Elder, 86, 96
Chaumette, Pierre-Gaspard, 141
Christian religion
  conformity to nature of, 28–
    29, 188

conformity to reason of, 31,
  41, 146
Christian societies
  superiority of, 13, 58, 98, 195
Chrysostom, Saint John, 155
Cicero, 5, 41, 51, 73, 86, 90
Civil Code, proposed, 34–41,
  55, 65, 87, 94–95, 99, 107,
  109, 114, 115, 137, 148, 149n,
  173, 177, 181
Clarissa, 25
climate, doctrine of, 25–26
Clovis, 68, 69, 74
Codrus, 86
Collet, Pierre, 159
commerce, 115
Condillac, the abbé Etienne
  Bonnot de, 10, 17, 18, 29n, 49
Condorcet, Marie-Jean-Antoine-
  Nicolas de Caritat, marquis
  de, 62, 87
Corneille, Pierre, 24
Costobarus, 83
Council of Trent, 99, 158
Crusades, 25n

Delille, the abbé Jacques, 24
democracy, 31–32, 38, 39, 55,
  69, 85–87, 101, 105, 106
Descartes, René, 18, 24, 197
Dionysius of Halicarnassus, 90,
  177
divorce
  effects on:

children, 38, 65, 110, 122, 186
marriage, 140, 144, 185–186
paternal authority, 38, 68, 95, 106, 108, 130, 148, 183–184
women, 38, 108–109, 176, 183, 186, 187
see also repudiation; separation
Domat, Jean, 197
Domitian, 90, 191
Dorat, Claude-Joseph, 24

Euripides, 87

fanaticism, 51n
Fénelon, François de Salignac de la Mothe-, archbishop of Cambrai, 24, 197
Flora (Roman goddess), 96n
Frederick William II, 103
French Revolution
origins of, 11–12, 101, 141

Gronovius, 87
Grotius, Hugo, 193
Guérin du Rocher, Fr. Pierre-Marie-Stanislas, 157

Helen of Troy, 88
Helvétius, Claude-Adrien, 17
Herod, 83, 191
Hillel (rabbi), 82
Hobbes, Thomas, 6, 30n, 67
Holbach, Paul-Henri-Dietrich Thyry, baron d', 14
Horace, 92
Hosius, Stanislaus, 154
Hume, David, 19, 25, 126n, 137, 140, 188

ideology, 24
impediments to marriage, 63, 155–159, 161, 163–164

inamissible justice, 30n, 101, 133
infanticide, 68, 88, 92, 99, 134
innate ideas, 13

Jerome, Saint, 89, 154
Jesus Christ, 57, 74, 83n, 93, 95–98, 102–103, 134, 147, 154
Jiménez de Cisneros, Francisco, Cardinal, 28
Josephus, 81, 83, 95
Julian the Apostate, 90
Jurieu, Pierre, 9, 30n
Juvenal, 89n, 95

Kant, Immanuel, 30n
Karlstadt, Andreas, 103

La Fontaine, Jean de, 32
language, theory of, 44, 48–52, 59–60
laws, theory of, 36, 51, 53, 71–74, 174–175
Le Brun, Charles, 24
Le Brun, Pierre, 118
Leibniz, Gottfried Wilhelm, 10, 24, 30n, 71
Le Nôtre, André, 24
liberty
among Christians, 27, 52
literature, 24–25, 31, 143–144
Livy, 89
Louis the Debonair (Frankish emperor), 68
Louis XIII, 69
Lucretius, 86
Luther, Martin, 8, 27, 30n, 35, 101–103, 123, 135, 137, 139
Lycurgus, 8, 87

Malebranche, Fr. Nicolas, 24, 30, 99
Maleville, Jacques, marquis de, 173, 177, 192
man, definition of, 15, 44
Marat, Jean-Paul, 141

marriage, 35–38, 62–66, 109, 175–177
Martial, 96n
Milton, John, 193
Mohammed, 8, 27, 57
Molière, 117n
monarchy, 39, 55
monogamy, 97, 110
Montesquieu, Charles-Louis de Secondat, baron de la Brède et de, 6, 8, 58, 68, 69, 84, 88, 90–91, 99, 106, 119, 191, 193, 196
Montmorency, Henri II, duc de, 69
morals compared with laws, 111, 149, 168, 187, 194, 195–197
Moses, 93, 98, 102–103
Müntzer, Thomas, 103

Naaman, 82
nature
  idea of, 10, 12, 14, 71, 97, 175
  of man, 36–37
  opposition of to the social and artificial denied, 10, 37, 71–73
  state of nature, 7, 10, 12
  see also Christianity, conformity to nature of
Necker, Suzanne Curchod, 84, 91, 119, 126, 136, 145, 188
Nougarède de Fayet, André-Jean-Simon, baron, 52

order, 27, 97, 99, 187
Origen, 154
Orléans, Louis-Philippe-Joseph, duc d', 173

Paul, Saint, 15n, 46, 59, 72, 74, 93, 103, 147, 154
Peter I (tsar of Russia), 68
Petronius, 95

Philip of Hesse, 103, 123
Philip II Augustus, 74
Pius IV, 154
Pius V, 154
Plato, 24, 55n, 86, 95
Plautus, 89
Plutarch, 90, 191
Poland, 61, 68, 75, 122–123, 153–165, 191
polygamy, 61, 62, 79–80, 92, 95, 123
Portalis, Jean-Etienne-Marie, 41

Quintilian, 71

Racine, Jean, 24, 143
Racine, Louis, 24
Radziwill, Barbara, 153
Rastignac, the abbé Armand de Chapt de, 82, 113n, 153, 161
Reformation, 13, 34, 99, 101, 139
repudiation, 74, 80–84, 88, 97, 99, 102–103
  difference between divorce and, 83–84, 90, 108, 190–191
  rarity of among simple peoples, 81–82, 89, 141–142, 167–168, 187
Richelieu, Cardinal de, 28
Robespierre, François-Joseph-Maximilien-Isidore, 141
Romulus, 90, 91
Roucher, Jean-Antoine, 24
Rousseau, Jean-Baptiste, 24
Rousseau, Jean-Jacques, 6, 7, 9, 10, 11, 13, 14, 20, 27, 32, 37, 47, 49, 51, 69, 70–72, 74, 146, 196

Saint-Lambert, Jean-François, marquis de, 15n, 24, 44, 100–101

Saint-Pierre, Jacques-Henri-
   Bernardin de, 183
Salome, 83
Ségur, Louis-Philippe, comte de,
   104
Seneca, 89, 191
sensations, doctrine of, 30
separation, marital, 95, 105,
   120–121, 141, 177, 178
   a mensa et a toro, 81, 103,
   177
Sigismund II Augustus, 153
similarity between domestic and
   public society, 38–39, 61, 68–
   69, 75, 77, 85–89, 97, 105,
   107, 122
Sixtus V, 28
social contract
   existence of denied, 55, 108
Solon, 8, 86, 134, 191
Stahl, Georg Ernst, 15n, 44n
state of nature, *see* nature

Stör, Thomas, 103
Suetonius, 95
Suger, the abbé, 29
suicide, 102

Tacitus, 11, 33, 50, 70, 95, 120,
   141, 177
Target, Gui-Jean-Baptiste, 189
Tarquin, 86
Tartars, 76
Terrasson, the abbé Jean, 173
Theophylactus, 155

Valerius Maximus, 90, 92
Valerius Publicola, 88
Verres, 9
Virgil, 176
Voltaire, 24, 27

Weiss, Franz Rudolph von, 124–
   125